Street Corners, Strangers, and Drugs

A Las Vegas Paramedic's Story

Lynn Mayers

ISBN: 1512084913
ISBN 13: 9781512084917
Library of Congress Control Number: **XXXXX (If applicable)**
LCCN Imprint Name: **City and State (If applicable**

This book is dedicated to my family, my friends, and all the wonderful people I have worked with in the past 22 years. The names used in this book were used with their permission.

CONTENTS

INTRODUCTION

"What's the grossest thing you ever saw?" asks the young teen as his small group of friends gather around the paramedic crew. "Have you ever seen a dead body?" comes from another young man. "I have seen quite a few dead bodies," says the paramedic. "The grossest thing...that's hard to say." Images of past calls flash through the paramedic's mind. The ambulance crew tells the youngsters that they have to go. They continue to push the gurney, loaded with equipment, to the patient's apartment.

Most people have developed their image of a paramedic's job from watching TV, a movie, or from personal experience. What is a paramedic's job really like? What kind of people do they see? What kind of health emergencies do they encounter? If someone really wants to know, they need to ask someone who knows firsthand. A realistic look at a paramedic's job would demand an uncensored look into the calls to which they respond.

So now, let's bring in the real side of paramedicine. Nothing would be more real than the actual written accounts taken from the journals of a real-life paramedic. That's where I come in. I have never studied literature or ever dreamed of being a writer. To explain how this endeavor came to life, I will take you back to 2003.

On April 4, 2003, I decided I needed to express my frustrations on paper. Back then, I called my journal my "paper psychiatrist." As a divorced, middle-aged woman with four children, I really needed to "talk" to someone about all the turmoil in my mind. As time went on, I recorded many of the bizarre, unusual, funny, touching, and sad calls that I had at work.

I started working for an ambulance company in 1992. Several years later, they were bought out by another company. Currently, I am still working part time as a paramedic.

I want to share with you some of the more interesting calls that I recorded. They are taken directly out of my journals with only a few changes made. Names have been changed or deleted. Hospital names have been given alphabetical designations. The street names and city areas are real. In Las Vegas, knowing the general location of a call paints a better picture.

Along with sharing many of the calls I had at work, I am also including some of the weird stuff from my personal life.

Being a paramedic has opened my eyes to many of the

wonderful and heartbreaking things that happen to people in this life. I have learned a lot about different kinds of people. Most of all, it has given me an opportunity to help people and show that I care.

As you are reading, remember that this book is not a literary effort to show my talent as an author. (Ha! I am silently laughing to myself.) This book is a sharing of human life, emotions, joy, heartaches, trials, and laughter.

CHAPTER ONE

ASSAULTS, SHOOTINGS, AND STABBINGS

4-29-03, 10:18 a.m.

Last night, we had a call for a man who was assaulted. Our patient was six-one, 212 pounds, not bad looking, was over at Shady Acres mobile home park (a real dive!). He had been drinking. He was hit in the head, near his right eye, with a bike peddle (crowbar per him). Two hours later, 911 was called. His right eye was swollen shut and he had dry blood on the right side of his face with fresh streaks of blood dripping off and on from his eye.

We've had so many assaults with similar-looking injuries that we didn't know it was as serious as it later turned out to be. We took him to hospital B instead of the trauma center.

After writing my report, we cleared hospital B. We transported our next patient to hospital B, also. Our previous pt had a CT scan, X-rays, etc., showing he had a serious eye injury. The globe was probably ruptured. An eye specialist came to hospital B and chewed us out for not taking him to hospital C. OK, fine! We ended up taking our assault patient from hospital B to hospital C operating room waiting.

Our assault patient really took a liking to me. "You're so beautiful. Can I have your phone number?" and on and on! He said, "I would crawl on my hands and knees for a mile through broken glass to hear you fart in a walkie-talkie." I asked him if he'd ever used that line before. No, he just made it up. He kept going on and on. He said I was the first beautiful woman he'd seen since he broke up with his girlfriend three days ago. I already told him I don't give patients my phone number. I didn't tell him my last name either. He wanted me to call him so he could take me dancing when this was all over.

Monday, 7-7-03, 7:46 a.m.

Right now, I'm drinking a diet cola and munching on reduced-fat potato chips. I'm trying to ignore the cookies that are "calling" me! "I can't hear you!" Last night, for our first call, we had a thirty-five-year-old man who shot himself in the abdomen (epigastric area) with a .22 caliber gun. He was complaining numerous times that his back hurt. Sometime during the ordeal I said, "Well, you SHOT yourself!"

We had an eight-to-nine-minute Code 3 transport back to trauma, but the telemetry wasn't done until about one minute out. The doctor chewed out FD [fire department]. I started pissing and moaning to a couple people near me. "I'd like to see him go out in the field and see what it's like!"

Wednesday, 7-23-05, 7:58 a.m.
I'm not going to write any dumb, goofy things this a.m. Last night, our first call was for a stabbing. It was near Simmons and Vegas area. When we pulled up, there were several Metro cars. As we walked up to the house, we saw FD inside and they canceled us. Metro standing outside said she stabbed herself right in her heart. "She's dead."

Sunday, 11-23-03, 12:22 a.m.
Why do people do some of the stupid things they do??? A fifty-two-year-old man sent his kids to a friend's house for the night, killed his wife (shot her through the chest), and then shot himself in the head. When we got there, we had to hold back for Metro. While we were waiting, we got a page that Metro wanted us to block off the end of the street with our ambulance. So we did that for maybe ten minutes. While we were sitting there, we could see several Metro cars and FD four to five houses down. Finally, dispatch cleared us to go in.

The house had a fence around it with a locked gate. I had to climb over the fence. When I entered the bedroom (FD and Metro already in there), a small, naked woman was lying supine on the bed—dead. The fifty-two-year-old man was lying on the bed with his legs hanging over the side. There was a bullet hole on both sides of his head. He had agonal respirations and a heart rate of 130. FD tried to intubate him on scene while I started an IV. He ended up getting intubated at the trauma center.

I called later and talked to a nurse at about 10:10 p.m. The man was put in trauma ICU [Intensive Care Unit], still with pulses and a blood pressure. She said his brain was "mush." They'll probably end up harvesting his organs. That reminded me, when I was doing my clinicals for paramedic school, I watched a doctor "harvest" a dead woman's corneas (for a cornea transplant). It was pretty interesting.

Saturday, 1-24-04, 4:28 p.m.

Last night, we transported an intoxicated twenty-one-year-old female from the Palms hotel to hospital A. Security there usually takes patients out of the crowds to the pool area outside. The patient was out there with several security guys. FD wasn't there yet and someone asked if we needed them. Not trying to be funny, particularly, I said, "Yeah, they can carry our bags." Was it the way I said it? I don't know, but that just cracked up the security guards. It was one of those "you had to be there" things to appreciate it. One of the guards said that was the funniest thing he'd heard in a long time. And to top it off, by the time FD got there, we were ready to go. And they picked up our bags!

On the way to the hospital, I was in front driving. As I was turning left from Flamingo to Maryland Parkway, an SUV going westbound tried to turn right in front of me (I had the green arrow). I quietly said, "What the hell?" He honked at me. He then went behind me, passing me on the left, honking, speeding toward…hospital A, maybe?

As I pulled into hospital A, I was wondering if we would see that car. Sure enough, it pulled up, crooked, in the little street next to ambulance parking. Several people got out, including a young lady holding her side. My partner asked them what was going on. "She's been shot!" My partner went over to enter the code to let them in.

Turned out she was in the back right seat of the car as they were in a club parking lot, leaving. A bullet entered their car and hit her (twenty-five-year-old female) in the chest. It went through her right breast near her nipple, out the underside, and into her rib cage. That was just before 4:00 a.m.

We waited with our patient for about an hour and later ended up transporting the injured female to the trauma center. She was awake, oriented, and complaining of right-side pain. The hospital staff were concerned that the bullet might have nicked her liver.

Comments: Let me explain something. Except for a very few incidents, I have really enjoyed working with the fire department. The men and women of the fire departments in Las Vegas have always been friendly with me and treated me with respect. And I treat them the same way. I consider them my friends. So, I can tease my friends, right?

Saturday, 3-19-05, 8:47 p.m.

I just put on the movie *Daredevil*. I think I'll put this (my journal) away for a while and watch it. Then I need to catch up on some interesting calls. (Hours later, Sunday, 3-20-05, 12:43 p.m.) Of course, interesting to us (EMS people) would be terrible for most people.

As we were driving to a post on the west side, we heard a crew get a call for shots fired. Hey, we're closer! We got on the radio and told dispatch where we were, so they gave us the call. By the time we got close, it was Code 4 [all clear]. The FD rescue intermediate was standing outside. He said it was a home invasion. A young woman was shot in the chest two times and was dead on scene. I said, "Ugh, that sucks!" Then a police officer and the FD paramedic came up and told us the real story. A young woman high on meth got into an older couple's apartment, had a knife, and the man shot her. "I don't feel sorry for her now!"

Saturday, 4-30-05, 6:50 a.m.

Yesterday, my partner called off. I worked eight hours with one guy, then did the FTE [field time equivalent] thing, driving around to the hospitals (of course, with the music cranked up), by myself, picking up backboards.

For the last about one and a half hours, I worked with another female paramedic. We transported a patient to hospital B. While my partner was inside finishing her report, I was outside enjoying the early morning (6:00 a.m.). I noticed three helicopters flying around in circles over downtown. What are they doing? They looked like Metro. Later, I found out a lady was driving south on I-15 just south of the Spaghetti Bowl when someone opened fire on her car. They shot several times into the passenger's side and left a big hole in the rear right window. The car, of course, went out of control and hit the median. She was killed. I've never heard of anyone being killed (shot) on the freeway here. Why was she shot? We may never know.

Last night, we jumped two calls because we were closer. The second one ended up being a twenty-seven-year-old male who was stabbed seven times: three times in the back, once in the right axillary, twice in the right elbow, and once in the left elbow. Ended up with a right hemothorax. He said he was "jumped from behind, didn't know who they were." Man, do you think Metro is stupid? Bad drug deal?

Tuesday, 8-23-05
Our next call was even more interesting. Fight in an alley behind the Stratosphere. When we got there, several Metro…

(Saturday, 8-27-05, 3:53 a.m.)…cars were in the alley. Two men were on scene. One had blood smeared here and there on his body and an abrasion on his face. My partner was checking him out when FD said, "There's someone else over here!" The two firemen were standing between two cars parked closely together. I told my partner I'd go check it out. There was a man lying on the ground between the cars. He had blood on his face and FD said he was stabbed in the neck. Then they opened his shirt, and there was a deep open laceration on his left chest. He was a goner! One of the firemen asked to borrow my stethoscope. No lung sounds. Duh! He's dead! The sheriff was on scene and found the body because he saw the bloodstains on the pavement where the assailant dragged the body. When we put the gurney away, we found more bloodstains on the pavement behind the ambulance that led to a small pool of blood in the gravel, evidently where he was stabbed. My partner said he saw the long knife, still wet with blood, on the hood of the patrol car.

Thursday, 7-24-08, 1:48 p.m.
(Transported someone to hospital) When we got to the hospital, I saw several police cars and an ambulance in the visitors' parking lot. Someone's car was parked in the ambulance parking area. Evidently what happened was this: Nurse went out to her car and found a dead dog and a dead man between two cars. She jumped in her car and drove the short distance to the ER. She reported it and then the police came. She was so upset she started throwing up. The man shot his dog and then killed himself. Some of his brain matter splattered on another nurse's car. Why did he have to kill his poor dog?

Thursday, 7-7-11, 6:04 p.m.
Last night at work started off with a bang! Got a call for a GSW [gunshot wound] in the Charleston/Fort Apache area (west side). When we pulled up, a young man was lying supine on the grass near the sidewalk. Metro and FD were on scene. We came from a ways off (not unusual), so FD already had an IV started. The patient, a twenty-year-old man, had a GSW in his left arm just below his left shoulder. The hole was just about a half inch in diameter—not much

bleeding. FD figured the bullet just stopped in his shoulder.

After we got him in the truck I noticed a small hard lump just below his mid left clavicle. And there was a slight swelling in his left upper chest area. By the time we got to hospital C trauma, the swelling in his chest had increased. He had no breathing difficulties. Looked like the bullet (small caliber) traveled through the soft tissue between his shoulder and chest and stopped below his clavicle. Probably also did some damage to his humerus. He told me he was driving to his girlfriend's house and a guy pulled up next to him, shouted, "Do you wanna die tonight?" and then shot him. It was an unfortunate incident, but he was lucky it wasn't worse.

When we got to the trauma center, it was hopping! There was a funeral at a mortuary for a young man who was killed last week. Some guy opened fire on the crowd and hit seven people. Four were transported by ambulance and three showed up at another hospital in private cars. Then they were transported from there to hospital C trauma. As you can guess, there definitely were gang issues going on there! A lot of the people hanging around the front of the trauma center were wearing red T-shirts.

Thursday, 1-26-12, 10:48 a.m.

Monday night, we transported six people. Five in a row were my patients. We had a call for a stabbing at a North Pecos address. As we entered the apartment complex, FD and Metro were on scene. A police officer was pulling the yellow Do Not Cross police tape across the parking lot. He didn't wait for us to go by with our gurney, so we had to go under the tape.

The patient, a thirty-nine-year-old man, was sitting on the sidewalk next to the apartment building. FD was holding a dressing around his left forearm. This guy was stabbed four times in the left leg, once in the left forearm (the biggest laceration about two inches long), and once just above the left flank area.

He spoke mostly Spanish. My seven years of Spanish (seventh grade–college) helps me a little at work, but I don't have the vocabulary I need for a lot of the situations we have at work. I was a little puzzled why he was stabbed so many times. Did someone hold him down? Did he offer no resistance?

A fireman rode in with me to hospital C trauma center. I started an IV and did telemetry while FD checked vitals and put him on the monitor and oxygen. His lung sounds were good, so I don't think the knife hit his lung. FD had already put an occlusive dressing over the stab wound on his back.

CHAPTER TWO

DRUGS AND DRUNKS

4-13-03

Three days ago, a sixteen-year-old, drunk, combative, foul-mouthed female bit me on my right arm. It made a deep indentation and later looked like a bad hickey. It's still bruised and a little sore. I really didn't think I needed to, but everyone said I should get it evaluated. So I did. Got a tetanus shot and was put on an antibiotic.

Saturday, 5-31-03, 4:34 a.m.

Our last call was for a 408 [drunk] male downtown. He was handicapped and used a walker. His injuries were from an MVA [motor vehicle accident]. Security said he kept falling. By the time we got there, he could barely sit on the pavement, kept falling over. He tried to spit on Metro, called us names, and gave security the finger.

Several weeks ago while at CC [Clark County] detention center, we ran a call with a man wearing a spit sock [mesh cover over head]. We asked Metro if we could have a couple.

Last night, my partner put her spit sock on our obnoxious drunk. When we took him to hospital A, we sure got some reactions! We had to wait in the hall for two and a half hours for a bed. One of the doctors came into the hall, stopped in his tracks when he saw our patient. Almost everyone who walked by made a comment. Of course, to complete the scene, the patient's arms were restrained to the gurney.

In his slurred, drunk voice he called me a "bitch" several times. The Metro bike cop was a "queer fagot." Etc., etc. It's hard to have compassion for someone like him. I hate taking drunks to the hospital just because they drink so much they can't walk.

Thursday, 9-18-03, 9:02 a.m.

Next day, Tuesday, we ran a call on a twenty-eight-year-old woman who ran into a Stop sign in the parking lot of Suncoast Casino. She was sitting on the grass next to the car when we got there. FD and Metro on scene. She was lethargic, mumbling incoherently off and on, pupils about 2–3 mm, and an initial heart rate of 160.

The car wasn't hers and a bottle of Xanax was found in the

car that belonged to the car's owner. The woman had blue residue (same color as Xanax pill—eleven missing) on her lips. We got her into the back of the ambulance. After I started an IV, I decided (fortunately) to restrain her arms and legs. At this time, she was mildly resistant to painful stimuli.

On the way in, for a couple seconds, I tossed around the idea in my mind whether or not I should give her Narcan. It wouldn't affect the Xanax, but maybe she has something else on board. After 2 mg Narcan, her pupils blew up to 5 mm, she became very agitated, started sneezing, and the incoherent mumbling increased. Possible addiction to narcotic pain killers? I usually give only 1 mg Narcan if I suspect a reaction like this.

Overdoses are one of my favorite types of calls. I also like 32B (or C)—unknown problem, unconscious. Let's see, I kind of like breathers, too. The two calls I hate the most are chest pain and MVAs. So many of the chest pain patients appear in no distress and nothing shows up on the monitor. Of course, we have had a good share of serious MIs [myocardial infarctions], but those are few. And another patient, probably the one I detest the most, that I truly dislike is the intoxicated man who wants to go to the hospital.

Thursday, 9-25-03, 7:21 a.m.
We also had a call with FD for a nineteen-year-old man huffing paint. Man, the odor was strong upstairs and he was spaced out. He was A&O [alert and oriented], but "high" on the fumes. When Metro got there, they decided to just give him a citation.

Comment: Maybe you could call this ironic, but just as I started typing the last entry, my chest started hurting. I think the incident is mentioned later, but I truly believe I messed up my lungs from exposure to aerosol hair spray. A couple years ago, I suddenly started getting chest pains at work and then the coughing started. It's better now, but I use an inhaler once in a while. I am using an Albuterol nebulizer now. So, the moral to the story is, be careful to what you expose your lungs. Even the everyday products can cause long-term damage. If only I could turn back time!

Saturday, 11-29-03, 9:30 a.m.
Wednesday night, we had a call for unknown problem (32B), male found down in closet, turning purple. We found a male (purple? I

couldn't tell) lying supine in the closet, head in the doorway. He had snoring respirations—about 12–16/minute. His oxygen saturation was 79 percent room air.

I placed a non-rebreather 15 liters oxygen on his face. Then I greased up an NPA [nasopharyngeal airway] with lidocaine gel. Stick one of those in a patient's nose and it helps open the airway, keeps the tongue in place. I barely got it stuck in his right nare when it caused a reaction. Prior to that he was out, with pinpoint pupils (typical narcotic overdose).

He reached up for the NPA, and I grabbed his hand. Then he became combative. Two Metro officers were standing there and came down on him. After a brief struggle, they subdued him. My poor partner was in the corner of the closet (small walk-in) trying to keep out of the way. I grabbed her arm and helped pull her out. Well, we never got a chance to give Narcan. Maybe I'll try an NPA on my next narcotic overdose! This patient, a man in his thirties, denied using any drugs and Metro couldn't find anything in the apartment. The previous weekend, he was with a known heroin user.

Tuesday, 5-18-04, 9:36 a.m.

Early Saturday night, we transported a thirty-nine-year-old man who was drunk and passed out in the casino at the Stratosphere. His only problem was he drank too much. He was in and out of it. We took him to hospital C.

To my "delight," while I was sitting at the stop light at Charleston and Martin L. King, on my way home, guess who walked in front of me on the crosswalk with a soda, eating from a bag of nuts! Yup! I couldn't help but think "You are a waste of our time and money!"

We have a new frequent flier who was transported one day last week three times to hospital D. We ran on him that third time. He still had his name band on. So we took him back to hospital D. One or two days later, we ran on him again. This time, he was only two blocks from hospital D, but he wanted to go to hospital C. He was so drunk, on the way in he forgot he chose hospital C and said he wanted to go to the same one (hospital D). Then he started with "I think I'm having a heart attack. My chest hurts." Oh, just shut up (didn't say it out loud)! I warned him he better stop crying wolf, because if he ever really has a problem, no one will believe him. Of course, I knew he either didn't hear it or didn't understand it. I might as well be talking to myself!

Wednesday, 7-7-04, 3:49 p.m.
I woke up a little early (had my alarm set for 5:00 p.m. I now work 7:45 p.m. to 7:45 a.m.). I think I got a little too warm. It's supposed to get to 107 today. Gotta love Las Vegas! Last night, we ran a call for a fifty-three-year-old homeless man who was walking out in a field, looking for his cat, tripped on some barbed wire, and probably fractured his ankle. His wife was with him.

We got him on the gurney, wheeled him across the dirt twenty to thirty yards and loaded him in the ambulance. His wife wanted to come, too, of course. I hate letting homeless relatives or friends ride up front. We have to sit up there, too! I looked her over real quickly when she had her back to me—she didn't look too filthy. She didn't smell too pleasant, though. Still, I let her ride in the ambulance.

She had a big, orange, convenience store plastic mug with her in a plastic sack. On the way to the hospital, she fell asleep. Then she dropped the mug on the floor. OH, MY POOR NOSE!!! At first, I thought it smelled like warm fermented orange juice. Then it got worse. After the call, we cleaned it four times (bleach, alcohol, disinfectant wipes, water hose) and it still stunk. Later, I sprayed it with an orange-scented room spray and covered it with a towel.

We had to apologize to the next couple riders. From now on, we check the drinks someone brings on if it's questionable. Of course, no alcohol! It was probably warm beer. It smelled like nasty yeast for a while. And no intoxicated homeless people up front. And if someone homeless sits up front again, I'm covering the seat with a sheet!

Thursday, 9-30-04, 9:08 a.m.
Last night was a very slow night. We had two transports. First was a thirty-nine-year-old lady who had a large boil on her back. She bumped her back against a wall and the boil ruptured. Yuck! White fluid oozing, well actually, more like dripping. And it stunk. We took her to hospital F.

Then we had an intoxicated, filthy, dirty thirty-one-year-old man who was sitting on a bus stop bench at Tropicana and Jones. He started to get up and took a nosedive on to the pavement. A couple young men across the street saw him and crossed the street to help him sit back up on the bench. It took them a couple minutes to get across the street (traffic lights). They said no one at the bus stop was willing to help him. We transported him to detox.

What a laugh! I wonder how many or what percentage of the people who go to detox actually detox off their alcohol or drugs and go "straight."

After we transported the second patient last night, we posted at 16I—an indoor post near Ann and 95. We were there from 11:15 p.m. until 7:00 a.m. Nap time, man! That was unusual!

Friday, 10-29-04, 9:13 a.m.

This week sure has been one for drunks! Tuesday night, our first call was for a drunk sitting on the pavement in front of the MGM. He drank a fifth of whiskey and was barely talking. We got him to take a few steps with assistance. We (especially my partner) wanted to take him to detox. I kept thinking, "I don't know. I think he's a little too intoxicated." My partner was in back and kept trying to keep him awake en route to detox, flicking his ears with his fingers...More later. I'm tired...

(Saturday, 11-6-04, 11:33 p.m.) When we got to detox, we got him to sit up and move to the foot of the bed. He had trouble moving his feet, so he was unable to stand to get out of the ambulance (patients have to walk into detox, with assistance if needed). I told my partner that we were going to have to transport him to the hospital. Then he started vomiting on the bed and floor. Even with us holding his head up, he had trouble throwing up. He was so drunk that when he threw up, he couldn't clear the vomit out of his mouth. He started making gagging sounds and his face started turning blue. We scooted him back while he was still sitting up. We were holding on to his head and suctioned his mouth.

We ended up calling another unit. I tried a couple times to intubate him. Then the intern (from the other ambulance) put a combitube down. I think our patient aspirated some vomit. I wondered later if we had taken him to the hospital if it would have been worse—lying on a bed, not being watched as closely, then vomiting.

Sunday, 7-15-07

Friday, we went downtown to CCDC [Clark County Detention Center] for a male with chest pain. He was a tall, handsome man. After he got on the gurney, he said he remembered me. I transported him about four years ago. When we got to hospital C, I was talking to him while my partner was giving a report to the charge nurse. The patient said when I previously transported him, I gave him a lecture about using drugs. I suppose drugs had been a leading cause for the condition he had back then. I don't get preachy with my patients, but sometimes I do "lecture" them like I would a friend. He said he actually stopped using drugs for a couple years. He seemed like an intelligent man (midforties), so maybe my friendly advice was taken to heart.

Several nights ago, a middle-aged man fell "asleep" behind the wheel at a stoplight on Rancho. As we pulled up, we saw one Metro patrol car pulled up nose to nose to his nice SUV. Another was right behind him. And another parked nearby. A Metro convention! They were all standing around. "We can't wake him up." I asked, "Did you pound on the window real hard?" All the doors were locked. It probably was a silly question and that's why they ignored me. Or was it because these cops (and they kind of fit the image) were "too cool" to pay attention to some female paramedic.

Then FD rescue pulled up behind us. The captain (I assumed), a tall, husky guy, went up to the window and pounded hard several times. Without even flinching, he reached into his pocket, got out his handy little tool, and gave the window a hard thump in the lower corner. Shattering, but still in one piece, the glass came crashing down to the pavement. The driver still didn't wake up. Oh, yeah, he was breathing. Metro said, "No, don't wake him up yet!" One officer pulled out a camera and took a picture of him through the windshield. Then the captain shook him awake. Someone is going to jail and getting a DUI [driving under the influence]! I have little sympathy for anyone who drives a vehicle after drinking alcohol.

Wednesday, 5-6-09, 10:26 a.m.
Last night, we had a forty-two-year-old female who went up to the wrong house and was knocking on their door. This was after midnight, so I bet she woke the residents up. Well, they called Metro and then we showed up. She was acting like she was drunk—unsteady gait, slurred speech, confused, and dozed off in the ambulance. She was wearing only a bathrobe and one slipper.

When we got her in the ambulance, we noticed she had some patches on her chest. My partner asked her if she is wearing a pain patch. I put my reading glasses on so I could read the writing on the patches. There were five 100 mcg Fentanyl patches taped to her chest with some clear tape! Normally, someone would wear one patch for seventy-two hours. After I got out of the hospital (October 2005 to January 2006), I wore one patch (50 mcg, I believe) on my upper arm. No wonder she was out of it.

She had a lot of what looked like burn scars on her right leg, hip, and stomach. She said she had a hip operation, but it was really a skin graft. It didn't look very recent. I wondered if she was prescribed the Fentanyl after the initial burns. We gave her 1 mg (half the normal dose) of Narcan to try to bring her around a little more. Her respirations were a little slow, too (10–12/min). When the Narcan started to take effect, she yelled, "What did you give me?!?!?" She got really agitated, trembled occasionally, was upset, sneezed a little, and moaned. Yep, she's addicted!

I tried to go off Fentanyl cold turkey a couple times. My withdrawal symptoms felt like what restless leg syndrome must feel a little like. But I was also upset emotionally. To finally get off the Fentanyl, I replaced it with Oxycodone (which I was also taking) and gradually decreased that amount.

Tuesday, 5-3-11, 9:18 a.m.

At work again, sitting at Sahara and Rancho (writing on paper to tape into my journal later). Last night, we had a call that came across as a man not breathing. He was inside a green car parked in front of a 7–Eleven. Oh, great, we are going to work a code! Then I thought, "Maybe it will be an overdose like the man who was in a fast-food parking lot…"

(Friday, 5-6-11, 1:55 a.m.) We're posted in an outlying area (Farm and Durango), so we may be here for a while. To continue the previous entry—"…shooting up heroin." Our current patient was a thirty-year-old man who was in the car with his brother. His brother said he just passed out. He pulled him out of the car onto the pavement and started doing chest compressions. When we got there, FD was already there, had an IV going and had given him 2 mg of Narcan. The patient had been in a car accident a few years ago and was still taking Lortab for back pain. He would take five to six 10 mg Lortab every day. Wow! So, this time he took several and drank a lot of beer. Stupid! Almost killed himself. FD said he was breathing maybe three times a minute when they first got there.

Wednesday, 1-2-12, 12:36 p.m.
Had two interesting calls worth mentioning. The first one was for a twenty-four-year-old male who went outside and smoked some Spice [powder sold by smoke shops under the pretense of using as incense or whatever. The labeling states do not use for human consumption]. My partner told me it's illegal now.

The patient's sister went out to the backyard and saw him and screamed. Her husband came out and found him bent over, on top of the air-conditioning unit, whole body seizing. He thought the patient was being electrocuted, so he kicked him off of the unit. Then they called 911.

This kid was pretty alert when we got there. We recommended he go to the hospital. He probably had a seizure. He got on the gurney and we brought him out to the truck. But after my partner started an IV and we were about ready to leave, he told us he didn't want to go.

He had several minor abrasions on his body. I'm sure they were from his body seizing while being on top of the air-conditioning unit. He kept saying all this was because he hit his head. Clueless.

I don't know what is in Spice, but I'll just call it "poison." If it can make someone have a seizure, it doesn't belong inside a body.

We had him sign AMA [Against Medical Advice] and then I went back to the house with him to explain to his brother-in-law why he wasn't going to the hospital.

CHAPTER THREE

ISN'T THAT SWEET?

Comment: This chapter was supposed to be about accidents, but I'm not in the mood to type about depressing things. So, let's cheer up and read about the lighter side of being a paramedic. It isn't all icky guts and gore and depressing, you know!

4-5-03, 3:36 a.m.

I just got home from working an eight-hour overtime shift. On the way to work, I heard a thumping sound from the back of the car. My right rear tire has a slow leak. I've been putting air in it every two to three days. I forgot to check it tonight.

So I pulled over (at Bonanza and Mojave). Fortunately, there was a convenience store (well-lit place) at the corner. As I started to change the tire, a man (family looking) in a nice van pulled up. He said, "I know it sounds sexist, but do you need any help?" I said no and thanked him. I've changed a lot of flat tires (especially last year). I continued. Then a young man walked up and asked if I needed help. No, thanks. I'm OK. He insisted! So I stepped back and let him take over. He was very nice. His friend walked up and talked with him as he was doing it. I graciously thanked him and he left. I really didn't need any help, but it's nice to know there are some gentlemen around willing to help the "weaker" sex!

4-27-03, 1:32 a.m.

Why do I always write in here when it's the wee hours of the morning? Thursday night, we transported a man from hospital B to his apartment on South Casino Center. I was driving. When I came to the intersection of Charleston and Casino Center, three motorcyclists were in front of me at the red light. One guy got off his bike, turned toward the ambulance, bowed down several times (bending at the waist, arms stretched out in front of him) and pointed toward me. I pointed back at him, waved, smiled, and quietly laughed to myself. I had a smile on my face for several more blocks.

Tuesday, 6-24-03, 2:20 p.m.

Last night, we responded to a call with a fire department engine. Joe [name changed] was there. I hadn't seen him for probably six months. Outside the house, he came up to me and gave me a rose (from the patient's garden) and a big hug.

Comment: Aaah! See? I told you the firemen were my friends!

Thursday, 9-25-03, 7:21 a.m.
Last night, we had a call for a man who had a dizzy spell while sitting at the table drinking milk. When we got there, he was feeling better and refused transport. He had a previous episode of vertigo and this felt similar. He is seventy or so. His son was standing by the doorway. He was handicapped, had trouble speaking and had a brace on his left leg. He said a few things to me. I listened intently because it was difficult to understand him. Then he asked if I could move our equipment so he could go through the doorway to the living room. I moved FD's oxygen tank. Then the son (thirty to forties) said to me, "Every time my eyes look at you they dance." I said, "Aaah" and gave him a soft pat on his shoulder. Then his father said, "Everything I know I learned from him." People can be so sweet and funny sometimes!

Thursday, 10-23-03, 8:32 a.m.
A couple weeks ago, one of our patients called the supervisor to compliment us on our compassionate treatment. I'm usually nice and caring with all my patients, but few of them go to any extreme to show their appreciation. One couple left a large platter of brownies at the station for us.

Friday, 4-16-04, 10:07 a.m.
Monday night when I went in for work, I checked my mailbox. When I opened an envelope that was in there and saw what it was, I said, "Holy crap!" out loud. Mr. and Mrs. ____ sent me a thank-you card with a $250 check in it. My partner and I transported him a couple months ago. I think it was for a respiratory infection. My partner was in back with him. He is seventy to eighty years old, owns a taxi/limousine company. He still goes to "work." I'm going to send them a thank-you card with a letter of appreciation. I called my partner Tuesday night before going to work to tell him to bring his mailbox key. When he saw his check, he was so overwhelmed that he got tears in his eyes. So far, from patients, I've received tips

of $100 (from a Japanese high roller), $10 from a patient's son, big plate of brownies from a couple, and now this. Today, I would be broke if it wasn't for him.

Comment: Technically, we are not supposed to accept tips from people. I have graciously turned down some people, but there are times when it would be rude to do so. The generous Oriental gentleman is one example. Security on scene told us not to turn down his gift. It would have been an insult.

Thursday, 7-30-09, 1:15 p.m.
Last night, ran a call for a sixty-four-year-old male with hematuria and abdominal and flank pain. On scene, I was standing next to the fireman. Then realized it was Neal [name changed]—British-type accent, cute, used to have a crush on him. He said, "Hi, haven't seen you for a long time." Gave me a kiss on the cheek. Aaah! Before he left, he gave me another kiss on the cheek and I kissed his cheek. I told my partner that was the most excitement I've had in months and months! Of course, I know that's just his way and he really doesn't mean anything special by it.

Comment: To any women reading now, yes, there are plenty of cute wonderful firemen and police officers out there! I have had my fair share of crushes, but we need to be professional as paramedics.

Saturday, 12-12-09, 9:10 a.m.
This last week I ran a call with a city fireman who asked how I was, hadn't seen me since my accident, and said he prays for me every day. I was really surprised. If he was actually telling me the truth, that is unusually amazing. He seemed like a really decent, honest man and I believed him. There are a lot of wonderful people in this world.

Comment: I'm sure there are many more sweet, funny stories from the last nineteen years, but I just didn't write them down.

Saturday, 5-17-14, 3:25 p.m.
This chapter would not be complete if I didn't include what happened to me while I was in rehab.

For about three weeks (in December 2005), a large group of

people (from two different ambulance companies, fire department) did an extreme makeover on my house. I'm not sure whose initial idea it was, but my house sure needed it!

I was allowed to leave the rehab for a few hours on Friday, December 23, to view my "new" house. The following is taken from an entry in my journal on Sunday, 12-25-05.

At 2:00 p.m., I rode over to my house in the ambulance with Mom and Dad...The first thing I saw when they opened the back doors of the ambulance was about three news cameras pointed at me. My friend, Denise, was standing there, teary eyed. I was wheeled into my "new" house on the gurney. When we got to the kitchen, I was surrounded by about six to eight news cameras. I had three mics put on my shirt and then a lady asked me questions. I answered some of her questions, then just started talking on my own, telling them about my accident, etc.

Then I got in my wheelchair and looked around the house. Doesn't even look like my house! It looks like a model home. Tile (nice!) in the living room, dining room, kitchen, bathrooms, and hallway. New cabinets in the kitchen, marble countertops in the kitchen and bathrooms. They all did an absolutely beautiful job! New furniture, new water heater, new landscaping.

Then before I left (to go back to the rehab), I opened presents and shed a lot of tears of joy over my "new" house. These people are so terrific!

All the news channels had a story about me. I must have been on TV Friday night for quite a few minutes if you put all the stories together.

On Saturday, I had to call the fireman who was basically in charge of the makeover (about the water heater). He told me I made the front page of the newspaper. What??? Front page? One of the nurses' stations had a copy of the paper and they let me keep it.

Thursday, 9-11-14, 2:39 p.m.
I just finished reading through all the pages of this book, looking for typos and other mistakes. I had scribbled a note on the first page that said, "Did you include the jacket washing?" No, don't think I did. So, here goes. Many years ago, during the winter, we responded to a call at one of the hotels. The patient decided to go to the hospital. We were all in the elevator when the patient projectile vomited on my jacket. Gross! The sweet fireman took my jacket back to his

station and washed it for me. Wasn't that nice? And, dear fireman, if you're reading this, I thank you, again!

CHAPTER FOUR

ACCIDENTS

Wednesday, 9-24-03, 10:42 a.m.
Monday night, we had a call for an auto-ped on Serene and Eastern. En route, I was thinking, "Yeah, a stupid parking lot 'Oh, my neck hurts' accident." As we pulled up, it started looking more serious, and it was in the street. We got out, grabbed the gurney, and walked up to FD who was by a man lying supine on the pavement. I could see immediately that he had bilateral tib/fib fractures. When I saw that, my opinion of the call changed! He also had femur and hip fractures. FD transported that patient. We transported another man who complained of right knee pain and back and chest pain.

It turned out the patients were two of four LDS [Latter-day Saints] missionaries who stopped to assist someone with car problems. A truck coming from the east hit both the missionaries. The first one (with multiple fractures) was thrown about sixty feet and the other about twenty to thirty feet. It was about 10:00 p.m. and they were probably on their way home when it happened. The first missionary is lucky he wasn't 419 [dead]. Years ago, a retired police officer from California and his wife were crossing Tropicana and he was hit and thrown about sixty feet, too. But he died.

Thursday, 4-22-04, 11:10 a.m.
This morning, about 5:00 a.m., we were headed to our first indoor post of the night. We were stopped at a red light on Flamingo and Arville. We were in the middle lane going west. All of a sudden, we heard a loud scraping noise and a motorcycle on its side came sliding by us to our right, sparks flying. It stopped in the middle of the intersection. I asked my partner where the driver was (I was driving). He saw him tumbling on the pavement and landed near our front right tire.

I put on the emergency lights. As we got out, the driver got up and walked toward his bike. He was drunk. He lived nearby and just wanted to get his bike and go home. He had road rash on his inner arms, a hole in the knee of his pants, and road dirt on his shirt. Fortunately, he was wearing his helmet. And it was a good thing no one was going through the intersection the other way!

A couple patrol cars and a motorcycle cop showed up. Not all of them stayed (the cute bike cop stayed—of course I noticed!). They gave him a choice: go to jail or go to the hospital. We all tried to get him to go to the hospital. Jail might not like taking someone who had been in an accident. The patient absolutely refused to get in the ambulance. He couldn't afford it. We tried. My partner gave him a good lecture, but it didn't sink into his intoxicated brain. All he saw were $$$. So, off to jail he went. The officer wanted us to fill out a statement because we saw the accident. I had my partner do it because he saw it better through his window. Not a good day for the motorcyclist. Sorry, but I don't have much sympathy for anyone who drinks and drives. Any adult should know better!

Monday, 9-6-04, 1:55 a.m.
Wednesday morning, a little after 2:00 a.m., we got a call for a thirteen-year-old boy who was dirt bike riding with his father. They got separated and he had been missing since around 7:00 p.m. Tuesday night. The Metro Search and Rescue helicopter had been looking for him for several hours. They almost gave up and then found him in a twenty-foot-deep ditch. From what we could see, he had abrasions and bruises. No serious injuries. But the news sure made a big deal about it. A news crew was on scene and did some videotaping. That morning, three TV channels ran the story several times, making a big deal of a kid and his father dirt bike riding or should I say "trespassing" on BLM [Bureau of Land Management] land! So, my partner and I were on TV. They showed us walking by with the gurney, loading the kid, and they showed a butt shot of me. The editor must have fallen asleep! For the next couple days, we had several people making comments to us about seeing us on the news. When I called home at 6:00 a.m. that morning to make sure Evan was up (for school), I asked Tyler if he could tape it. He got three or four different stories.

Tuesday, 6-7-05, 9:37 a.m.
Oh, and I will never buy an SUV! A lady in her late-twenties was driving a Pathfinder, probably a little too fast, west on Spring Mountain Road. She looked down, probably fiddling with something, and ran into the rear driver's side of a full-size truck. Smash-a-roonie!!! Her car flipped over on its roof and skidded down the street about thirty yards. She only got a few scratches, fortunately, because she was wearing her seat belt. The guy in the

truck was OK. I could smell some alcohol on her breath, even over her perfume.

Thursday, 6-23-05, 9:41 p.m.
Wednesday morning, at about 4:30 a.m., we were heading to post (29G) via the airport tunnel. My partner was driving.

"Did you see that truck in the gravel up against the wall?" No, I didn't. I was tired and starting to doze off a little.

We were heading west and turned around at Las Vegas Boulevard. If you're going west on Russell and turn left toward the airport tunnel, there's a short (two to three feet) concrete wall (parallel to the road) with gravel on the other side. Then there's a large concrete wall to the right of the road (perpendicular to the road) where the tunnel begins. Sure enough, an intoxicated (five beers) twenty-five-year-old female, going too fast, missed the turn, flew over the short wall, and smashed her Toyota Tundra (large truck with extended cab) head-on into the wall.

She got out of the truck, and when we got there, she was standing at the short wall (three to four feet from her truck). When I walked up to her, I saw blood on her hand and sleeve. "Are you OK?" Her right leg hurts and it's numb. Her pant leg was torn.

We put a C-collar on her and lowered her on the backboard down to the ground. As I started to cut her right pant leg, I saw a lump protruding, covered by her sock, from her medial ankle. Crap! She has an open fracture. Also, a large laceration across her right knee, hidden in her fat (she weighs 240 pounds, five feet four inches tall). She also had a jagged, large laceration on her left leg. I had to cut her right shoe and sock off. Her tibia was dislocated and sticking out about two inches.

I told my partner I couldn't carry her (my end of the backboard) ten to fifteen yards down gravel to where the wall was only about one foot tall. It was three to four feet tall where she was. FD took several minutes to get there after our arrival. We had to wait for them. After FD got there, they helped us lift her over the wall right where we were and to the gurney.

At the hospital, X-rays showed a fractured fibula, and multiple (two?) fractures of her right midfemur. Her right thigh had a large bruise and the thigh had increased in size.

Tuesday, 8-23-05

Sunday night, my partner got an intern. A very young man from Utah. We didn't have any interesting calls on Sunday, but last night was much better. I got to work a little earlier (about 18:57 for 19:15 shift) than usual to be able to adhere to the "ten-minute rule." The crews are supposed to be ready to go ten minutes after their scheduled shift starts. It's usually hard because there is almost always something missing on the truck.

We were almost ready when we got a call at 19:20 to Calville Bay. Good thing my partner knew where it was. I figured, "Lake Mead...drive I-95 to Boulder City..." Nope. You take Lake Mead Drive in North Las Vegas all the way east.

Our patient had a waterskiing accident. They didn't have any details for us, so our imaginations were conjuring up scenarios. If he/she was very serious, the helicopter would probably have been called.

When we got to the dock, the boat was just pulling up with a man on a backboard on the deck. The accident occurred as he was trying to get up on a wake board and twisted his left leg. His feet were secured in the boots (or whatever you call them) so that probably contributed to his injury. The crew on scene already gave him 5 mg of morphine, and on the way in, I gave him another 10 mg. Not much relief with the movement of the ambulance.

10-17-05
Read the chapter titled "I Don't Want to Die Tonight." This incident really sucked and changed the rest of my life!!!

Sunday, 5-27-07, 7:23 p.m.
Yesterday on my way home from a doctor's appointment, I witnessed an accident that seemed like a movie scene. I was driving north on Martin Luther King Boulevard toward the entrance to I-95 southbound. Just before turning onto the freeway entrance, I glanced ahead of me. There were several vehicles under the I-95 overpass. All of a sudden, in front of a vehicle in the inside northbound lane, a big splash of water shot up about ten feet. A small car flew up into the air, turned upside down, and came crashing down on its roof. The car in front of me pulled up to the group of cars and numerous people got out. I stopped just before the freeway entrance and called 911. They answered very quickly. The operator said, "They're on their way." I debated for a couple seconds if I should stop and check

it out because I'm a paramedic. There already were a lot of people out and about. They didn't need any more cars clogging up the scene and FD was already on the way (FD station is very close), so I decided to keep going. What could I do anyway? On the way home, I kept thinking, "I should have stopped. I should have stopped!" What if they tried to move the patient and compromised a possible spinal injury. Aaah!! When I got home, I told everybody about it and was still thinking that I should have stopped. I won't do that again. Someday, it might actually make a difference.

Comment: I have stopped several times when I have witnessed accidents. All those times my medical knowledge didn't make any difference. I was just a witness.

Thursday, 12-9-10, 8:39 p.m.
The last two nights at work seemed to last forever! When it felt like 2:00 a.m., it was only 10 or 11:00 p.m.! And we were pretty busy, too. At the end of the shift this morning, we were at Rainbow and Russell. We cleared to go home and I drove to Tropicana and Rainbow to gas up. Our truck used unleaded fuel only.

I pulled up to the gas pump and saw a Metro officer walking up to my window. Figured he was just going to say hi. He asked, "Are you here for our girl?" Evidently, she went into the convenience store bathroom, locked the door, and passed out on the floor. Metro wanted us to check her out. I called dispatch and said we were going to look at her. I had heard them dispatch the call to someone else, then they gave it to us.

(Friday, 12-10-10, 2:00 p.m.) To continue, we checked her blood pressure, pulse, and blood sugar. It was all fine. I asked her if she had been drinking. She didn't seem real drunk. Her car was there and had some front-end damage—quite a bit, but not massive. She didn't need to go to the hospital and I believe Metro was going to let her go. They "knew" she had hit something, but couldn't prove it. Then surprise, surprise! A tow truck pulled up with two cars on it. And he had her bumper inside one of the cars! Well, sorry, sweetheart, here's Metro's proof. She's going to jail for hit and run! I looked over at her and she knew she was in trouble. I couldn't hear her, but saw her say, "#!&#!"

Friday, 5-27-11, 4:50 p.m.

Last Thursday (19th), we had a call for a "man down" on the travel lane, northbound I-15. That can't be good. We were the first EMS unit on scene. A man, forties to fifties, was lying prone, head to the right, on the pavement. There was a small amount of blood (about 50 cc) under his head that appears to have dripped down from a spot on his forehead. He was apneic, pulseless, unconscious, and unresponsive. He didn't have any gross, noticeable traumatic injuries. He was wearing long pants, but it looked like he might have some left leg fractures. The way our new protocols are, he needed to have injuries incompatible with life, lividity. Asystole used to be one of the conclusive signs. My partner asked about putting him on the monitor. I really didn't think it was necessary, but I said, "Sure, why not?" He was in asystole. His pupils were fixed and dilated.

It always seemed weird to me that almost everyone who gets hit by a car, with any force, loses their shoes. His shoes were several yards from where he was. The small truck that hit him had a good dent in the top of the hood. FD was talking to the poor driver that hit the man. He was complaining of some chest pain.

Saturday, 1-5-13, 9:49 a.m.

Another interesting call we had on New Year's Eve showed how dangerous it can be for someone who has seizures to drive.

About 2:00 a.m. we got a call for traumatic injury. It was at a car dealership. When we got there, the patient was standing outside with Metro. He was complaining of neck pain—very tender to palp. He also had some right elbow pain (abrasion) and some minor abrasions.

The gate to the back lot was busted open and his car (a small convertible sports car) was way down by the wall (forty to fifty yards). There was debris in the back lot and some cars were definitely out of place.

The police officer walked down to the patient's car and took pictures. Then he showed them to us. Totaled! Air bag deployed, windshield shattered, and a mangled mess of metal. He was by himself in the car, fortunately. FD said that if his girlfriend had been riding with him, she probably would have been killed.

The last thing our patient remembered was traveling north on Mojave, going about thirty-five mph. Mojave comes to a T at Sahara and then there is an entrance to the dealership. What apparently happened was he had a seizure, probably stomped on the accelerator, sailed across Sahara, crashed through the gate, hit several cars, then smashed into the wall. The patient didn't think he hit the wall because the car wasn't up next to the wall. Well, at an increased rate of speed, the car hit the wall and bounced back a bit.

Comment: Today is April 6, 2015. I wasn't planning on adding any more to my book, but the next call is a bit of a doozy, so I just have to put it in here. Due to my financial situation, I went back to work full time on January 1.

Wednesday, 1-28-15, 8:12 p.m.
I have been meaning to record some calls I went on this month. Due to procrastination, I don't know the actual dates, but I guess it doesn't matter.

We got a call for an MVA on the southbound off-ramp from I-15 to Silverado Ranch. We were already on South Las Vegas Boulevard, so we continued to Silverado Ranch and then west to the freeway.

As we approached, we saw a small white car in the middle of Silverado Ranch, at the end of the off-ramp. It was facing northbound. Nothing impressive. A female NHP [Nevada Highway Patrol] officer walked up to the ambulance and told us he's dead and she needs us to pronounce him (officially say he is dead).

We got out and walked over to the car and saw the other side. Oh, my! Unbelievable! The whole driver's side from the front bumper to the rear was sheared off! A young man (midtwenties to early thirties) was sitting in the driver's seat, his left leg hanging out and his torso and face facing outward. His left forehead had a hole in it the size of a half dollar. The edges of the hole were jagged with several cracks extending outward about an inch.

I really didn't need to, but I checked his pulse and his pupils. He was pulseless and had dilated pupils. There were clumps of what was presumably brain matter in the backseat. He did not have his seat belt on.

Near the end of the off-ramp was a little traffic island with a large light pole at least one foot in diameter. There were scrapes on the right side and a tiny bit of blood and tissue.

Evidently, he hit the pole at a high rate of speed (I'm guessing at least eighty mph) and the pole sliced through the car from front to rear, about as far in as the outside edge of the driver's seat. I wonder if he had had his seat belt on if this would have had a more favorable outcome for him.

CHAPTER FIVE

CARDIAC ARRESTS

Saturday, 7-19-03, 2:40 a.m.
This week has been a strange one for calls. Tuesday, we had several interesting calls. Call for a seizure in a taxi. When we showed up, FD had the patient lying on the pavement. As we stepped out of the ambulance, FD yelled "It's a code!" We shocked him three times while he was on the pavement. He was in fine v-fib [ventricular fibrillation]. Nothing! We loaded him into the ambulance. I intubated him and FD started a line and began drugs. Unfortunately, he didn't make it. At the end of the shift, my partner said that was the first time she's seen me intubate anyone. She complimented me. Said it was a smooth, good job. I was a little surprised. It was an easy intubation.

Thursday, 9-18-03, 9:02 a.m.
Monday night, our first call was for a forty-two-year-old man who was having sex with his girlfriend, finished, stood up, and then collapsed to the floor. The girlfriend supposedly did CPR [cardiopulmonary resuscitation]. FD said he was in asystole when they got there. They had the pacer pads on and were trying to intubate him when we got there. The man probably would not have survived, but...after looking at the monitor strip at the hospital, the initial rhythm looked more like fine v-fib.

Sunday, 10-19-03, 12:15 a.m.
Last night, we were posted near hospital N. We had a third rider, a young girl still in high school. We were sitting outside the Texaco store having a drink and a snack. It was pretty busy there. Friday night and "Hey, baby, let's hang out at the Texaco!" A lot of young kids were coming and going. A small group of kids (young teens) walked by us and a very friendly, perky girl said hi and then she asked if we've ever seen a dead body. I said, "Yes, a lot." She made some kind of icky comment and went in the store.

Saturday, 11-15-03, 3:38 a.m.
Tonight, we got one of the brand-new trucks! I was really surprised.

It had only 553 miles on it. Our truck the night before had more than 300,000. The new trucks are bigger, wider, taller, and sit a little closer to the ground. So jumping the median can't be done very often. The buttons up front are all different and the cabinets in the back are, too. The driver's seat is more comfortable.

Our first call was for a cardiac arrest. Wouldn't you know it, the first night I decide to wear my sweater, we get a cardiac arrest (I'm going to get hot!). An eighty-eight-year-old female evidently fell down the stairs. Her daughter-in-law came home and found her at the bottom of the stairs. When we got there, she had agonal respirations and a heart rate of 40. We got her intubated and gave atropine. She went into asystole. Some compressions and epinephrine and we got good pulses back. Hospital D was only three minutes away. They had gone on divert recently. I did telemetry saying, "I realize you're on divert, can you accept an eighty-eight-year-old cardiac arrest?" I really don't need to ask them. With a cardiac arrest, you just go to the nearest hospital. But I have heard crews say that they had been asked to divert from there with a cardiac arrest. They told us we would "be waiting in the hallway." Well, screw that! So we went to hospital N (another five to seven minutes away). They were actually closed (no beds available), but had a room available when we got there. The staff was a little pissy, questioning why we didn't go to hospital D. I told them what they told us. The reasoning behind my decision is that I have no doubt that hospital D would make us wait in the hallway. Their halls are usually lined with beds with patients on them. Hospital N does that also, but not as badly.

Comment: I am typing this on 2-14-12. Normally, I say "Bah, humbug" to Valentine's Day. Last night, I worked a shift from 16:30 to 04:30. On scene of one of our calls, I got a hug from the same fireman three times! Since I went part time I have missed that. Because my social life sucks, I tell myself that work is my social life. Having friendly attention from cute firemen doesn't replace a significant other, but it helps! And to all you firemen (and women) who visited me while I was in the hospital: Thank you so much! It meant a lot to me. I especially want to thank the Las Vegas Fire Department. You guys were terrific.

Sunday, 2-8-04

Monday night, I worked an OT shift. We got a call at the airport for a breathing problem. As we pulled into the south gate entrance (off Kelly Lane), we got a page informing us that the patient is unconscious, blood coming from her nose. What? The patient was in a bathroom.

We pulled up to a building with stairs on the outside going up to the second floor. A person was holding the door open, a couple people yelling at us to run—she's not breathing. We grabbed our equipment and walked fast. Running would save only a few seconds and put us in danger of falling or tripping with heavy equipment.

An overweight sixties-to-seventies-year-old (don't remember her exact age) female was sitting on the toilet and became short of breath. A family friend stated he found her slumped on the toilet. They moved her to the floor, on her side, and tried to clear her mouth. She had stopped breathing.

When we got to her, security was by her side, the AED [automated external defibrillator] on the floor. I couldn't tell whether it was attached. He said no shock was advised. On the way to the call, FD was in front of us, but didn't turn at the right spot. I said, "They must be going to a different call." Well, to sum up, we ended up working this call for several minutes by ourselves, with the help of bystanders, until FD finally got there.

I really don't like working cardiac arrests. My partner and I had one this week. A forty-seven-year-old male was having sex with his girlfriend. He became short of breath, was gasping for air, and then collapsed. When we got there, he was lying supine on the floor next to the bed—no CPR. The female on scene said he had been down only five minutes. He was in asystole. FD got there first. I let the FD paramedic completely run the call [give verbal commands] because he's a good paramedic. He had trouble intubating him. His partner got the tube. They also had a female intern with them.

On the way back to the hospital, I did the telemetry and did chest compressions while standing up. The fireman was sitting on the bench behind me, holding on to my belt (at one time my hips) so I wouldn't fall over. I had taken over compressions because he was dripping in sweat. I was warm, but not to the sweating point.

After we got him to the hospital, the doctor decided to defibrillate him. He was in asystole. Per our protocols, we don't shock asystole. The doctor said, "Shock anything." Another medic and I looked at each other. What??? I said to him, "Like in the movies! They always shock asystole!" They worked him for quite a while. Gave him more meds. I was surprised. He had already been down for almost an hour.

While I was in the break room writing my report, someone came in and said they did a pericardiocentesis and found out he had a massive heart attack. I then went out to get a nurse's signature. I passed by numerous family members standing near the room. The nurse told me the patient's daughter collapsed and went into v-fib. She was now in the room next to her deceased father. I wonder how things turned out for her. Next time I go there, I'll ask.

Sunday, 6-27-04, 12:21 p.m.

Right now, I'm sitting on my bed watching the tape that Denise and I made when we were working together on the Strip on 12-31-99. We were posted by the Mirage. Denise got a lot of pictures of the crowd passing by, sometimes coming up to the camera.

Now I'm watching *Liar, Liar* with Jim Carey. I've seen it numerous times. I need to catch up on my entries. I should be writing down a lot of my "different" work calls. I'll describe some of the calls I've been on lately.

9D [cardiac arrest] for a thirty-seven-year-old male on north 9th St. We had a third rider with us. When we arrived, a female in her sixties met us outside and pointed to where he was. "He's in there." We were at a one-story apartment complex. The door was open and I walked in to see a 250–300 pound male facedown on the couch. He had thrown up on the pillow and all over the end of the couch—a thin layer of dark-brown emesis. His underwear was pulled down to the bottom of his rear end. He had defecated. His right arm was hanging down toward the floor. I reached down and tried to move his arm. STIFF! This guy was dead!

A couple daily pill containers were on the coffee table and his prosthetic lower left leg was leaning up against the table. I told our third rider to feel the stiffness (rigor mortis) in his arm.

When Metro arrived, they went into the apartment and brought out his three roommates—pale, thin men. This place was a halfway house. I suspected they all had histories of alcohol/drug abuse. Obviously the "stiff" (not very respectful, huh?) had some serious health problems. Our question—and Metro's, too—was, why was his underwear pulled down? One of the officers asked how long it takes rigor mortis to set in. A couple hours? What exactly is it?

None of my medical dictionaries describe it very well, except "the coagulation of the muscle proteins" or the lack of ATP (adenosine triphosphate). I'm going to look it up on the i-Opener.

Saturday, 8-7-04, 12:22 p.m.
Thursday morning (at 6:02 a.m.), we got a call for an MVA at Flamingo and Buffalo. On the pager it mentioned car vs. power box. We were near Fort Apache and Summerlin Parkway. It took us about nine minutes to get there. En route, we asked dispatch if Nevada Power was en route to the call.

As we pulled up, the FD engine and rescue and Metro were on scene. FD was by the driver's door, had a seventy-five-year-old female patient on a backboard, C-collar in place, starting to bring her out of the car. We brought our gurney up to the patient and they slid her onto it. One of the firemen said, "I couldn't feel pulses." She didn't look good. Part of her face had a slight blue/purple tinge and I couldn't detect any respirations.

We were so close it took less than ten seconds to get her into the ambulance. My partner had already jumped in the back. I yelled (not real loudly) to my partner, "We've got a code!" I jumped in, he stuck an OPA [oropharyngeal airway] in her mouth, I checked her pupils, and put her on the monitor. She was in asystole and her pupils were fixed and dilated. There was no obvious trauma that would indicate a traumatic cause of death. If there had been, hopefully FD wouldn't have extricated her. But, anyway, I was really expecting to see some kind of rhythm on the monitor. Maybe PEA (pulseless electrical activity). She had the four presumptive signs of death (unresponsive, pulseless, apneic, fixed dilated pupils) and one conclusive sign of death (no electrical activity on cardiac monitor, i.e., asystole). Even if we didn't put her in the back of our truck, we would still have to put the monitor on her. No obvious trauma.

This morning, my supervisor kind of jokingly teased us because "we" put a dead body in our ambulance. I just looked at him and walked away! So what should we have done, huh? Leave her on the gurney outside on the street for all to see? Put the backboard with her on it down on the pavement? Screw that!

We had to wait on scene for the coroner and the mortuary people. The coroner and Metro agreed that FD "screwed the pooch." And another thing, the car was next to the power box that had live wires! FD should never even have touched the car!

Before the accident, someone driving in a car next to the patient's car saw her starting to swerve and then it looked like she passed out. Her car knocked over and scattered six newspaper stands. It also damaged a power box and a fire hydrant. The fire hydrant jammed under the rear of the car, finally stopping her.

I sat in the back of the ambulance with her, writing up my report, etc., for two hours! After that the coroner arrived and I watched him examine her. He explained that a white ring just inside of the iris indicates a heart attack. He rolled her over, and by then (two hours later), she had some serious lividity going on.

When the mortuary guys got there, they put the blue zipper body bag on the bench seat. We lifted her on the backboard to the bag and rolled her off the board. I've never seen a person being put into a body bag (the coroner already put a toe tag on her). I felt sad. This poor woman was alive just a few hours ago and now she's getting zipped up in a plastic bag.

Tuesday, 5-31-05, 9:50 p.m.
Thursday (or Friday), our first call was for a man down—Ogden and Maryland Parkway. When we got in the area, three kids (about ten to twelve years old) flagged us down. They showed us where this person was. There's a big dirt lot on the southwest corner of the area. At first, I couldn't see anything because of the weeds. As I walked closer, I could see a homeless man's "camp." Bedding was laid out in the dirt with some belongings scattered around. Lying on the bedding was a very *purple* man! He was dead! He looked like he had been sleeping with his arms bent, hands on his chest. Very rigored and profound lividity. The abdominal veins looked bizarre—very vivid and purple. My guess is, he fell asleep at night, died, and then "cooked" out in the one-hundred-degree weather all day.

Wednesday, 6-22-05, 8:28 p.m.
I'm always too tired after work to catch up on my entries. So here I am again at work, writing on paper that I'll have to tape into my journal. Right now, we're at 16I (Ann and 95 indoor post). *Gladiator* is on TV. Just started.

Last Friday, I worked an eight-hour OT shift. Our last call was one of those heartbreaking, "if-only" situations. A fourteen-year-old girl snuck out of her house to go ATV riding with her friends. This was about 2:00 a.m.! She fell off the ATV and became unresponsive, with only some moaning and slight body movement. One of her friends carried her back to his house. He said she fell off at about 2:00 a.m. They (including a male neighbor in his sixties) waited about thirty minutes to call us. She started vomiting and five minutes before our arrival, she stopped breathing.

When we got to the house, she was lying supine on the bedroom floor. No one seemed upset or excited. I passed the neighbor man (thinking he was the father) as I went through the front door. Two young kids were sitting in the room on the other side of the bed. The patient had pink frothy fluid in her mouth. I scooped it out of her mouth with my gloved hand, kneeling beside her. I glanced down at her chest and abdomen. She wasn't breathing. Of course, as soon as we walked into the room and saw her on the floor, "Oh, #!&#!" was my silent mental response. We got the call as traumatic injury, patient vomiting. Did not expect a code.

We started working her. Got her intubated, IV started, gave 1 epi and 1 atropine. In a couple minutes, we got pulses back (145, then down to 120s), but her pupils were fixed and dilated. Her lungs were very junky. Obviously, she had aspirated. FD got there first and initially I was saying do this, do that, like I was in charge. I realized quickly that I was probably stepping on the captain's toes, so I backed off verbally. The captain was busy setting up to intubate, so he wasn't talking much. I did compressions while my partner started the IV.

The captain thought we should take the patient to hospital C peds/trauma. We were probably five miles north of hospital D. Hospital C would be another eight miles on top of that. Nearest hospital, I said. The only obvious trauma she had was a large abrasion on her right hip.

Last night, we were at hospital D and asked about her. She died. If only they had called earlier, maybe she might still be alive. If only…

Thursday, 7-7-05, 2:56 a.m.
A couple days ago, we ran a call on an eighty-eight-year-old woman who has felt "malaise" for a couple days. She also felt a little short of breath and had a headache. Everything checked out pretty good. Last time, about two months ago, when she felt like this she was anemic. I told her we could take her to the hospital and they could

run some tests, blood tests. She said she'd rather wait until morning to see her own doctor. She said she just wanted to die. She was the youngest in her family. Everyone else is dead. She didn't seem overly emotional. She really meant it. She refused transport.

About 1:00 a.m., I got a page from dispatch to call another paramedic. That paramedic ran on our patient (after we saw her) at about 10:30 p.m. for cardiac arrest. She was in PEA. They paced her on the way to the hospital. When they transferred her over, the hospital staff took the pacer off. That was it. They called her shortly after that. Was the "malaise" her body getting ready to die? She got her wish. I wonder if we had taken her to the hospital, would she still be alive today? Sometimes when it's your time to go, that's it.

Thursday, 7-21-05, 4:27 p.m.

Haven't written in ten days! I'm sure I've missed a few good calls. Last night, we ran on a forty-four-year-old man with chest pain. He lived in an apartment complex, and when we got there, he was sitting outside with FD. He didn't look so good. He was diaphoretic and you could tell he was in pain. He said he had 10/10 midchest pain that started fifteen minutes ago while he was watching TV. The pain started in his back, then went to his chest. He said he had no medical history, didn't smoke, drink, or do drugs, except some marijuana in the past. He was five feet nine inches tall, about 180–190 pounds. I consider forty-four young, so in my mind I was thinking possibly it was respiratory. He did say that the pain increased when he took a deeper breath. He took an aspirin soon after the pain started.

We got him into the ambulance. I started an IV on him and made some comment about treating it as cardiac until proven otherwise. His rhythm was a little irregular (some PVCs [premature ventricular contractions]) and his T-waves looked a little elevated. When we did a 12-lead [ECG], the analysis was acute MI. Crap! The real thing! I gave him some sublingual nitroglycerin. It didn't change his pain at all. The FD paramedic was sitting in the truck with me. The patient said, "I'm not going to make it." I told him, "You'll be all right."

I looked at the monitor. Was that movement? No! He was in v-fib. I gave him a precordial thump and told my partner to grab the pads. We shocked him two times and then he came around. He was grabbing his chest and moaning. That must have hurt! I explained to him what happened.

To make it short, the doctor told him if he hadn't called when he did, he probably wouldn't be here. And we saved his life. He thanked us, and I told him he did a good job calling us so quickly. Just before we left the hospital, I was talking with a nurse who brought up his urine screen on the computer. It was positive for amphetamines and I think barbiturates, too.

Monday, 8-15-05, 4:08 a.m.
What an appropriate time to make this entry (408 means *intoxicated*). A frequent flier, homeless drunk, died yesterday at hospital B. He was found in an alley by a Dumpster. His heart rate was 180, blood pressure was 40/?, and his temperature was 109. Did the nurse really say 109? I was standing by the nurses' counter looking down at a 12-lead strip. I said, "That's not good!" She said it belonged to him. It was a wide complex tachycardia.

Sunday, 8-26-07, 5:52 p.m.
This week had some good calls. I only worked Tuesday, Wednesday, and Friday, but I'll get paid for taking Monday off (my birthday). Tuesday night, I worked with another paramedic. Our last call was for a cardiac arrest at the Wild Wild West hotel on Tropicana. My first reaction was that he'll probably be unworkable. A lot of the arrests in the early waking hours have been dead for a while. Family finds them not breathing.

This seventy-eight-year-old man came out of the bathroom clenching his chest and crumpled to the floor in front of his wife. Metro got to the room before us and the officer said the wife was making a panic-stricken attempt to do mouth-to-mouth. The officer was doing chest compressions when we arrived. My partner and I made a comment about doing at least one round of drugs on scene before we call it quits. But amazingly enough, the man was in v-fib and after three shocks and getting intubated, we got pulses back. And then he started breathing a little on his own! His pupils decreased in size from about 5–6 mm to 3 mm. We may have a code save!

At the hospital, he started having some purposeful movement in his extremities. That's a great sign! One of my first code saves as an intermediate started moving a little at the hospital (saw his feet moving). The police officer on the scene made a comment to me that every time he sees me I'm with a different partner. Since June 5, I've had about twenty-three different partners! Maybe my real partner will come back tomorrow.

Comment: I came back to work on June 5 after being out nineteen months because of my accident on 10-17-05.

Sunday, 10-07-07, 6:21 p.m.

After that call, we had one for a thirty-four-year-old male, unresponsive. They thought he took something. En route we got more info: "CPR in progress." Crap! It's a code.

When we got there, there was a large (about 330-pound) male lying supine on a water bed. Can't work a code with someone on a waterbed! So the firemen and I got him off the bed and dragged him down the hallway to a bigger area near the front door. Several police officers showed up, too. And the rescue paramedic called for the engine to come for lift assist.

FD intubated him. I got the IV and pushed all the drugs. His wife/girlfriend said earlier he had taken some morphine and Xanax. Later found out another lady (I think when they were at her house) gave the patient a methadone and Xanax pill. She also gave him a bottle with probably about thirty to forty pills (methadone and Xanax). She said he passed out at her house. I'm not sure exactly how he got back to his own house...or even if all this occurred at his house. Well, he went to sleep at midnight and his wife said he kept rolling over on her and was snoring loudly. Then he stopped breathing. 911 was (supposedly) called right away.

Something about this whole call didn't sit right. Had he been apneic for longer? How many pills did he actually take? He also had his own prescription for Lortab and Soma for back pain. He was incontinent of urine on his jean shorts. We gave him several rounds of epinephrine, atropine, some Narcan, and the sodium bicarb. He was pronounced dead shortly after arrival at hospital B.

Sometimes, I do mention it politely to people not to give anyone prescription meds that don't belong to them. I wonder how many times someone dies because they take prescribed meds that don't belong to them. I remember a man years ago who was prescribed methadone for shoulder pain. What? He didn't take an overdose, but almost died from respiratory arrest. Why would a doctor prescribe methadone for that? I'm not a doctor, but that didn't seem right.

Saturday, 3-22-08, 10:31 a.m.
Last Monday, we had a call at a dialysis center on Main Street. I didn't even know that place was there! The patient was a young man (age—what was it?—late twenties, thirties? Don't remember). The dialysis center called 911 because they couldn't do dialysis on him. His blood pressure was 250/150, he was vomiting, he wouldn't let them check his blood sugar, and he was fidgety and shaking his legs.

On the way to the hospital, I was in back with him. I got a blood pressure of 230/130, blood sugar read "HI," and his oxygen sats on room air were 79–81 percent. I put him on oxygen nasal cannula (NC) to start and got his sats up to 93 percent. I wanted to start an IV on him, but he said, "You won't find one. They have to do a central line." I asked him if he was refusing an IV now and he said, "Yes" (I documented that). OK, fine, whatever. I would have tried if he hadn't refused. Then en route, he pulled off his NC. I told him he needed the oxygen, but he said he didn't want it. Again I asked him if he was refusing and he said, "Yes" (and of course I documented that). He appeared alert and oriented, so I wasn't going to press the issue. If he was mentally altered, I would have restrained him to keep the oxygen on if I had to. Actually, I have to admit he kind of ruffled my feathers, so my attitude with him was "Whatever!"

Several days later, I spoke with the nurse who was in charge of him. She said while the central line was being put in, he went into cardiac arrest. When we transported him, he had a crappy rhythm, so I did a 12-lead on him. He had wide QRS complexes with elevated T-waves. He was a medical train wreck.

Comment: I don't remember if he survived and left the hospital.

Saturday, 7-5-08
A couple weeks ago, on a Monday, we got a call for a 9D [cardiac arrest] for a two-month-old. Initially, I hoped it was a false alarm. Maybe the baby was temporarily choking on milk and they thought he stopped breathing. I've had a few of those calls. Then I thought, "Crap! I don't want to work a pedi code!" When we walked into the apartment, the mother was sitting on a couch with an obviously dead (mottling from the chest and up, apneic, etc.) two-month-old baby lying on its back next to her and the older brother (five to seven

years old) on the other side. Cute little baby…dead…parents upset…the whole scene started getting to me. My eyes filled with tears. After the call, I told dispatch I needed a few minutes to recover.

Comment: Right now, the memory of that call is bringing tears to my eyes. I hate running calls like that one. If you ask a paramedic what the worst call is, many of them would say a sick baby call.

Tuesday, 1-12-10, 9:05 p.m.
Last night, we had a call for cardiac arrest for a fifty-four-year-old male. He was sitting on his couch, eating dinner. About an hour later, he got up, grabbed his chest, and collapsed. He went into cardiopulmonary arrest. He vomited sometime during the incident and aspirated. When FD got there, a family member was doing chest compressions. Fire said his mouth was full of vomit. The engine and rescue were both there, so there were about six or so firemen on scene. I helped the paramedic who was working on his airway. What a mess! We suctioned the emesis numerous times. After he intubated him, I started ventilating and said, "I don't see any chest rise." The abdomen wasn't moving at all either. My partner checked his lungs and said she heard lung sounds and no belly sounds. So I believed her. Shortly after, vomit started coming out of the corner of his mouth.

After we got to the hospital, my partner and I were in our EMS break room while I was writing up the report. I said, "I wonder if the tube was really in?" She went and asked the doctor and he said, "No." Crap! He didn't have a chance of surviving anyway, but if he had, that misplaced ET [endotracheal] tube would have screwed up his chance. I did notice that it was getting harder to bag (ventilate) him. The FD paramedic didn't seem too concerned. (He never found out the tube wasn't in.) This was all an exercise in futility. The man was down ten minutes prior to EMS arrival. Even though they did chest compressions, his lungs were probably full of vomit. If only he hadn't vomited, their CPR would have helped, it would have been easier to intubate him, and his chance for survival would have been better. I really should have insisted that he pull the tube because there was no rise and fall of chest with ventilations, emesis started coming out of his mouth, and it was getting harder to bag him. The FD paramedic made a comment that if the family wasn't there, he would not have worked him.

Comment: Medicine is called a practice because it isn't perfect! Even when a call for a cardiac arrest goes very smoothly, the chances for the patient's survival are slim. We do see people survive a cardiac arrest, but more often, it is not a positive outcome.

Wednesday, 8-25-10, 9:27 p.m.
Comment: This entry was written on a separate piece of paper while I was at work. Then I glued it into my journal.

We're at hospital H, waiting for a bed, with a patient who was wandering around a neighborhood claiming that he is God. Metro found a meth pipe on him and confiscated it. When we got here, the charge nurse informed us that they had no beds. So, we'll wait. I wanted to go to another hospital, but technically we can't bypass a closer hospital with a patient with altered mental status.

Our first call tonight was a doozy! The call was for a forty-five-year-old male who had multiple seizures. When we arrived, he was lying supine in bed, talking. Didn't seem postictal. The house was a place for patients to go after they leave rehab. This man had a stroke while in the hospital in April. Tonight, staff said he had a full-body seizure lasting 25 seconds, then another one 5–7 seconds long, during which they called 911.

FD had him stand up to take a few steps to the gurney. They were a little harsh on him when he had trouble walking. The patient had a stroke a couple months ago, so he had left-sided weakness. We got him into the ambulance. He was very sweaty and kept complaining of not being able to breathe. We had him on high-flow oxygen, but that wasn't helping.

I didn't like the way he looked, so I asked my partner to go to the hospital Code 3 (lights and siren). On the way in, the FD paramedic (who rode in with us) asked why we were going Code 3 for a seizure patient. After we got to the hospital, we were waiting for a bed with the patient still on our gurney. A nurse came over and gave him some Ativan to calm him down. Whoa! It sure calmed him down! He stopped breathing and went into cardiac arrest! We helped the hospital try to resuscitate him, but it didn't work. He died.

Friday, 5-27-11, 4:50 p.m.
Tuesday night, we had a call for a man who went into cardiac arrest on a bus. The bus was downtown. Someone said the man had a seizure, then went into arrest. The FD rescue and engine just barely beat us to the call. The man was lying on the floor of the bus. He still had some agonal respirations and was in v-fib. Rescue transported him to hospital B.

When we transported to hospital B on Wednesday, I asked the charge nurse what became of him. She said he became a coroner case because a white substance was found on him.

CHAPTER SIX

THE LIGHTER SIDE OF MY FAMILY

Comment: After that last chapter, I need a break from the heartbreaking side of being a paramedic. So now, for the lighter side of my children (Erin, Brianna, Braden, and Evan) and me.

5-6-03, 8:24 a.m.
Tonight, Erin, Brianna, and two friends of theirs did something that was really cute. They painted signs that said "I," "(picture of a heart)," "U," "(guy's name)." They went to where he works at a pizza place and attached the signs to their rear ends. While he (the guy) and all his coworkers were looking out the window, my kids and their friends turned around, bent over, and displayed their butt signs. Erin said he turned red. He gave Erin a couple hugs.

Monday, 12-8-03, 3:24 a.m.
Evan is reading *The Miracle Worker* (Helen Keller) in school. For an assignment he was supposed to be blindfolded for one hour. So last night at 9:00 p.m., he started. First, I had him brush his teeth, then go through the pile of his and Braden's dirty clothes in the bathroom and pick out his. He did very well for not being able to see! He felt for pockets, size, abnormalities, fabric. Then he went into the kitchen, poured himself a drink of water and poured me some diet cola on ice. Then we went for a drive around the neighborhood. I didn't guide him to the car. He felt the sidewalk edge. In the car, he could tell direction of turn and what street we were on. When we got home, he accidentally bumped Erin's glass of soda off the banister (by the front door) onto her lap. Then I asked Evan to find Paris (our dog). He was in the backyard. I was quite impressed with how Evan handled all that!

Monday, 11-15-04, 12:53 a.m.
Guess what? I cleaned up my bedroom! Yeah, I know! Miracles do still exist in modern days!

Monday, 2-14-05, 6:56 a.m.
On the way home, I got some Valentine's goodies to give to the kids. When I walked into my bedroom, there was a box of chocolates with a teddy bear, a sign saying "Mom" with numerous hearts on it (homemade by Brianna), and two shiny red metal roses on my bed. They also bought me a chocolate heart and put it on my bed a couple days ago. I ate the whole thing in one day.

Thursday, 6-23-05, 9:41 p.m.
At work again. This morning after I got home, Braden and Evan were still awake. They came out to the dining room and Braden wanted Evan to crack his back. Braden lay down prone on the floor and Evan pushed bilaterally on his spine. Sometimes it pops pretty good. Not so much this time. "Hey, do mine!" I said. So I lay down prone on the floor. Evan pushed once on my lower back. The response was a surprise to us all. No spine noises. Just a short, quick, moderately loud "fart." We all about died laughing. The boys fell onto the couches in the dining room, trying to contain themselves. I was still lying on the floor quietly laughing/crying. Tyler was asleep on the living room couch. We were trying not to wake him up, but he yelled, "Braden!" I got up and told Tyler it was my fault. It was one of those "you had to be there" moments to fully appreciate it. I don't know if I've ever heard the boys laughing so out of control.

Saturday, 3-4-06, 11:32 a.m.
Did I mention that a couple weeks ago, Tony Curtis talked in Brianna's class? She was so excited! Afterward, she got to hug him and had a picture taken. I talked to my mom on Thursday. She was jealous. He has always been one of her favorite actors.

Tuesday, 2-23-10, 11:47 a.m.
Comment: This entry was made a couple weeks after the death of my ex-husband.

Yesterday, I went to Walmart and on the way back, I started crying for a minute. I soon stopped myself. Crying doesn't help, it's not going to change things—those kinds of thoughts went through my mind. Shortly after I got home, Ava (my two-year-old granddaughter) woke up from her nap. I got her out of her crib and we were lying side by side on my bed chilling. My stomach growled and she looked at me and said, "You fart?" I lost it! I laughed so hard I lost control. And then I started crying at the same time. And then Ava moved the little blanket from the "fart area." I don't know what she was looking for. That was the best thing anyone could have done for me. I felt like a pressure cooker that had just released all its steam. I felt better for hours after that. It really is true that laughing is good for you. I'm sure a genuine smile helps, too. So, the cure or treatment for sadness is regular heartfelt laughter and the passing of time.

Thursday, May 13, 2010, 1:01 p.m.
Ava is really starting to talk. Several days ago, we were standing by the open front door (child gate across it). I pointed to my car and said, "Grandma's car." Then I pointed to my truck and said, "Grandma's truck." Her response surprised me. She said, "NO. Braden's truck." He drives it more than I do and she obviously has noticed that. I told Braden what she said and he laughed.

CHAPTER SEVEN

I DON'T WANT TO DIE TONIGHT

Sunday, 11-27-05, 9:04 a.m.
I don't believe I have written my account of what happened on October 17. So, here goes. Monday, October 17, it had been raining. Man, I hate working in the rain! I wore my rainy day hairdo (hair in ponytail, no bangs). My partner had an intermediate intern. We were just starting our shift, the rain had let up, and the intern was going to drive first. We received a call (at about 8:00 p.m.) to district 3325 (way down south like Wigwam and Maryland Parkway) for an eighty-two-year-old man who fell. I was sitting in the jump seat in the back. My partner was up front in the passenger's seat.

We were traveling south on I-15, got to about Tropicana, when the engine died. "What's going on?" "We lost power!" The intern pulled over to the left emergency lane. We got out, flipped open the hood and checked the oil. Dry as a bone! When we started the shift, there was a yellow post-it on the driver's window from the mechanic saying the oil, etc., was checked. We went to the back of the truck and my partner pulled out his flashlight and lit up the pavement behind us. Big oil streak behind us! Someone mentioned later that the new trucks, which we had, held a lot of oil.

I had made a comment sometime in this process that it was dangerous standing out here and we should get back in the truck. Before we had the chance, my partner and I were standing at the back of the ambulance. I was near the left driver's side of the bumper and my partner was standing closer to the jersey wall—about four feet tall. Next thing I knew, I was sitting on the pavement with a mangled left leg. It happened SO FAST! A car (small, like a Camaro, fortunately) spun out of control on the oil (and the pavement might still have been a little wet) and smashed into the back of the ambulance.

My partner was moaning, "My leg!" I felt like I was in a surreal world. It's hard to explain how it felt. I put my left hand under my left thigh. It was all wet. The intern called dispatch on the radio and told them what happened. She was OK. I had to lift my partner's left leg off my left leg. I asked our intern to cut my left pant leg. When she got to the knee I said that was enough. I could see my lower leg bending midshaft.

I remember her going to the front of the truck and I was shouting to her to get me the portable radio. I yelled it several times, but she didn't come with it. Later found out she couldn't find it. Somehow, I managed to get ahold of my cell phone. I called dispatch—BUSY! Dialed another number—BUSY! Tried a third time and someone answered. I told them we have a Code 5 (life and death) situation. "My partner and I have been hit by a car. We need NHP out here NOW to block traffic. I don't want to die tonight!!!"

About that time another car smashed into the "Camaro." Fortunately, it didn't move it. The "Camaro," so I heard later, hit the bumper of the ambulance and buckled it under. The bumper/fender is pretty big, like a step to get into the back of the truck. Now, I could hear sirens. Thank God!!

They got me on a backboard and I could feel them lifting me over the jersey wall as I was grabbing on to the holes on the outside of the board. I told them, "Let's get out of here!" I don't remember anything during the ride to the hospital. They said I cracked a joke or two on the way to the hospital.

The paramedic and his partner, along with a fireman, transported me to the trauma center. He said they started two large bore IVs, but they couldn't give me any morphine because my blood pressure was too low (systolic in the seventies). I remember when I got to the trauma center seeing Ann's (a nurse) face. I said, "Hi, Ann." I don't remember anything else. The paramedic said he didn't cut all my clothes off so I could have some privacy (save embarrassment). When the car hit me, it tore a large chunk of skin from my buttocks down. I had an open femur and tib/fib fracture. I had lost a lot of blood. I remember getting numerous blood transfusions the first week. They said a lot of my fellow colleagues showed up outside the trauma center that night, but the head doctor wouldn't let them in. I think finally a few people got to see me when I was in trauma ICU. I remember waking up with the Et tube still in my throat. Some of my family was there. I couldn't talk so I wrote on a piece of paper to ask or answer questions. I had a titanium rod with pins put in my femur and my tibia. Numerous staples were put up the side of my leg to bring the tissue together. Fortunately, the skin was in good enough shape to staple together.

Comments: I spent about three months in the hospital and rehab. Nineteen months after the accident, I went back to work. The injuries I already mentioned were minor compared to the complications that followed. Some of those were/are: traumatic blisters followed by tissue necrosis on my leg (resulted in scars and tissue and nerve damage), reaction to heparin (thrombocytopenia) which I believe caused a hemothorax (had three chest tubes and surgery), blood clots (some of which caused necrosis to two toes and resulting in partial amputation), arterial damage, venous stasis…to name a few. Getting hit by a car is a lot more than breaking some bones and tissue damage!

CHAPTER EIGHT

OOPS! GROSS AND WEIRD

Friday, 6-27-03, 11:11 a.m.
Wednesday night, we took a patient to hospital B. When we were finished, we drove over to a convenience store for a quick drink. Some new girl was there, so no free drinks. My partner and I got our drinks and got back in the ambulance. Our intern got in and said, "She charged me for my coffee!" I said, "That's because she's new." Then the door closed.

We went 10-8 (available), were given post 8 (Charleston and I-95) and started driving east on Charleston. When we were at about 15th Avenue, we got a page: "You're inturn (yeah, that's how they spelled it) is at station one." I thought, "They're trying to give us *another* intern? We already have one!" Then I turned around and looked in back. "He's not there!" "Dispatch, copy page!"

We went back to station and found our intern. At the convenience store, when he got into the truck, he was getting money to pay for his coffee. He didn't say anything about going back in to pay. We assumed he had paid when he first went in. When he came out and saw us driving away, he thought we were teasing him. But we kept going. He walked over to the station! He said he wasn't mad, and we said, "You'll laugh about it later."

Saturday, 7-19-03, 2:40 a.m.
We got a call for a man down—between the Olympic Gardens (a gentleman's club) and the doughnut shop, next to the magazine stand. As I was walking up to him, I thought he had vomited all over his face. Upon getting closer we realized it was poop! The man who called 911 saw the guy standing around earlier. Then he saw him lying down with a couple men hovering around him. They ran off, and he called 911. I guess they had defecated on his face. Several small lumps were on his face, on both eyes, his nose, and mouth. He was so drunk he didn't know what happened. I wiped off his face with 4 x 4s [gauzes] and a towel before I roused him. Yuck! When I told a nurse at hospital N the story, he "appreciated" it. "Maybe he should watch how much he drinks!"

Comment: Later, someone educated me about the poop incident. It's called a Boston steamer. Whatever!

Sunday, 11-16-03, 3:20 a.m.
Another eight-hour overtime shift. This time, I worked with one of my interns I had several months ago. We had only two transports—a slow night. While I was waiting at the station to go home, an EMT was telling me how FD and our company transported an over-five-hundred-pound patient from his rehab facility to hospital G (about six to eight blocks away). They pushed the patient's hospital bed down the street with the rescue, engine, and ambulance following behind. He said the ambulance crew refused to transport the patient on their gurney and FD wouldn't transport either. I've transported people weighing more than five hundred pounds before, but I guess this person's fat spread out a lot side to side. Wouldn't it have been funny if a news crew got shots of this procession!

Comment: I'm not sure what our supervisors thought about this. It was definitely out of protocol. Now we don't have this problem. We have a special bariatric truck equipped to transport larger patients. It has a larger gurney and a ramp and a hoist to pull the patient into the back of the ambulance.

Sunday, 8-29-04, 8:15 a.m.
Last night, Tyler told me something he heard on the news. A lady was sitting on her couch, heard the phone ring, and got up to answer it. There was no one on the line. But while she was up answering the phone, some idiot drove his truck into her living room and would surely have killed her if she had still been sitting on the couch. Was God calling her on the phone? Tyler jokingly said she should have dialed *69 to see who had called!

Wednesday, 10-20-04, 11:38 a.m.
Some recent calls: Got a call for an unknown problem, man in a Dumpster. It was behind a warehouse near Industrial and Sunset. FD drove up on a ramp near the large Dumpster and I parked near the bottom of the ramp. As we approached, a young man (early thirties) wearing a tank top popped up out of the Dumpster. On his head was a small light (not on right now) strapped to his forehead. He had a

bewildered, "Huh? What's going on?" look on his face. It was almost comical. My partner asked, "Whatcha doing, man—Dumpster diving?" "Yeah." FD looked at my partner. "You KNOW what that means?" My partner said when he was sixteen he tried living on his own and would Dumpster dive for food. This guy was looking for computer hardware, software, or whatever.

Sunday, 7-3-05, 1:39 a.m.
No really exciting calls to write about. Several mornings ago, while in the ready room, someone asked if I heard about an ILS (intermediate life support—no paramedic) crew going back hot to trauma. "No, what did they have?" Some guy stuck his finger into his eye socket and popped out his eye! Then he completely ripped it out. Ahhh!! "Why did he do that?" "God told him to!" The crew put his eye in a Styrofoam cup with saline water. Was someone off his medication? I know there's a scripture in the Bible about plucking out an eye. Let's see…Matthew 5:29 ("if thy right eye offend thee, pluck it out, and cast it from thee: for it is profitable for thee that one of thy members should perish, and not that thy whole body should be cast into hell"). Jesus spoke in parables and not everything he said was to be taken literally. I don't think he wants us to literally pluck our eyes from our sockets! Maybe this man's poor sick mind heard this verse before.

Saturday, 9-20-08, 4:15 a.m.
Midthirties-year-old male who lives in a dumpy apartment on 16th Street, drinks every day, abuses the 911 system, called earlier yesterday and went to the hospital. For what? I don't know. Six hours later…back home again, and he calls 911…again! After Metro arrived, we managed to talk him into going to detox. And the nice patrolman took him, instead of us taking him. Less than two hours later (just after 1:00 a.m.), we got a call for a man located around the corner from detox at the convenience store on Washington and Las Vegas Boulevard. It was him! He wanted to go to the hospital, but we wouldn't stand for that. FD called Metro.

While we were waiting for Metro to arrive, he changed his tune several times. "Can you just let me go?" He was sitting on the rescue's rear bumper. "I want to go to the hospital." "My back hurts." "My stomach hurts." Etc., etc.!

He was wearing only long pants. I felt a little sorry for him.

He wasn't very intelligent. Unless that was the alcohol talking. I don't think so. Was he deliberately abusing the 911 system? Metro checked him out and he had priors for system abuse. Metro said to us to either transport him or let him go. Metro believed because he already went to the hospital today, he had a legitimate complaint. I guess that was their reasoning. So we let him go. Shortly after he turned his back to us and started walking away, his pants made a comical parting statement. They suddenly dropped down to his thighs, showing his butt cheeks! It was a good laugh!

Friday, 9-25-09, 8:24 p.m.
Comment: The next story is a big oops. No one was injured, but it should never have happened!

Do NOT let your guard down! There are some procedures you must always follow because you never know when it will bite you in the butt if you don't. Last night, something happened because I let my guard down and didn't do what I always do.

We got a call to Charleston/Jones area for a possible psych patient. There was something in the notes about him drinking…was it Windex? And eating glass. Whatever! But, as usual, along with the notes on our computer, for this kind of call, it said, "Please hold short." If it doesn't, dispatch will send the message over on our pager. So, for these calls, we park at a safe distance from the call until the police clear us, telling us it's Code 4.

I was driving and we parked on a side street next to the shopping center where the patient was. After a couple minutes, I noticed the top of the fire department's engine, with its emergency lights on, parked in the shopping center. "Let's go check it out," said my partner. First mistake. It doesn't matter what FD is doing. If they want to run in before the police get there and possibly get shot at, that's their problem! Well, that's what I always think to myself when FD doesn't hold short.

But why was tonight different? So, I pulled up behind the engine. A fireman (with big muscular calves, wearing shorts, and my partner made a point of pointing out his physique!) climbed out of the engine and filled us in on what was going on. The patient was around the corner of the building throwing things around. Fire decided they were going to drive further across the parking lot. We followed them and parked facing away from the man.

My partner said, "Let's turn around so we can see him and watch him" (mistake #2). I turned the truck around and we could see him sitting on the pavement leaning against the wall. He stood up and shook his loose pants. "Looks like he's trying to shake a load loose," my partner said. Gross! I don't know about that! He didn't have a shirt on. He walked over to something on the ground, picked it up, and put it (his shirt) on.

Here he comes! He's walking toward our truck, nothing in his hands. "If he comes much further, I'm driving away!" I said. But I just kept staring at him, watching his body movements, almost mesmerized. He stopped at the front of the truck, bent over, and was staring at the grill. "What's he doing?" Of course that should have been a big fat clue that he was WEIRD! I could see my partner starting to reach for the air horn. I didn't say anything, but was thinking that wouldn't be very nice. Hind sight, I wish she had blasted him with it!

He walked around to my side and I thought, "If I just lower my window an inch, I can hear him and still be safe." "Do you have a light?" he asked. He pulled a cigar from above his ear. He was average height and build with hair down to his shoulders and some facial hair. He didn't look very intimidating. Ha! Weirdos come in all shapes and sizes. "No, I don't have a light."

I glanced forward for a second and in a surge of psychotic anger he reached up and jammed his fingers in the small window opening. He yanked back and forth on the window so violently that it rocked the ambulance. I was stunned! "Where's the window button?" raced through my mind. "Lynn, drive away!!!" my partner yelled.

The window crashed to the pavement and he stumbled back out of my view. I recovered from my three to four seconds of stunned disbelief and drove the truck about ten yards. Never in my seventeen years working for this company has anyone ever acted like this! We park outside at our posts and frequently have people walk up to the truck. For our safety (now I know better!), I lower the window only a tiny bit so I can talk to them. Never again!

Metro pulled up and ran and tackled him. They cuffed him and left him lying on the pavement. Later, my partner asked me if I saw him licking the pavement. What?

Right after I moved the truck, I called the supervisor. My voice was broken with emotion. The sup was relieved that it was just a broken window and we were all right.

After I filled out a statement, I walked over and looked at him. I was pissed! Mostly pissed at myself for letting all this happen. This was not like me. I am always careful about holding short. So, as I stood there looking at him, the natural reaction would be something like "You asshole!!!" and give him a swift kick in the stomach! But my usual emotional control prevailed and I said, "That WASN'T very NICE!!!" I was upset for hours, mentally kicking myself in the butt for letting something happen when I knew better.

At the end of my shift, I was talking with the sup and she told me this story (paraphrased): A college student was writing home to her mother. She met someone. She was in love. They weren't going to get married 'cause it's just a piece of paper. She was pregnant. She quit school and they were going to travel around the country. Actually, all of that was a lie. "I got a D in my class and I need money for books." So after reading the first part, the mother was so relieved that it wasn't true that she wasn't upset about the D or her daughter needing money. When I first called the sup and she heard the distress in my voice, she thought something really terrible had happened. Only a broken window! But I hate making mistakes and it takes a while for me to forgive myself.

Tuesday, 5-3-11, 9:18 p.m.

Last night, we had a forty-three-year-old female who Metro was called for because she was possibly soliciting. As we pulled up on scene, the fireman looked at us and shook his head. They had put their pulse ox on her finger and she took it off and stuffed it down her pants into her crotch area! You could see the cord hanging out of her pants. FD said she could keep it! Metro was standing several feet from her as she finished off her can of beer. She was something else! She was so outrageous it made us laugh. She was making sexual gestures, trying to grope us, and asking for kisses. Had to keep out of her reach! Needless to say, we had to restrain her extremities and put the torso straps on. The way she was talking, she seemed almost possessed. So, how would I describe her? An intoxicated (she had trouble walking), possessed, sexual deviant on drugs. She had a name band from hospital A on her wrist. So, guess who got our present?

Sunday, 9-30-12

A friend who used to work the same place I do came over to my house this afternoon. She asked me if I have any calls in my book from other people. After she told me about the following call, I had to include it in my "Oops" chapter. Here goes.

We got called to a 10D (chest pain) in an old part of town (built in the 1980s) with big houses and big yards. We arrived with a county engine on scene. The patient was sitting in the backyard by the porch. It was a summer day and they had a nice deep pool filled with water. We brought all of our gear: monitor, approach bag, and gurney. After assessing the patient, we found he was having a classic textbook MI (heart attack). He was cool, pale, and diaphoretic with elevation on his EKG. We started treating the patient. It was becoming a load-and-go situation (serious).

The fire captain turned and looked at me and yelled, "Where the #%#& is your gurney?" I turned and looked at him and said, "Why the hell are you yelling at me? My bed is right here!" I turned around to look for my bed and it was gone.

My gurney had rolled off into the pool and was in the deep end. I said, "Look, there it is!" He got mad, turned red in the face, and stormed off.

We had to call another ambulance to transport the patient. We used a pulley from the fire truck to get the bed out of the pool. We had a neighbor boy jump in and attach it and we pulled it out.

After the call, we had to 10-19 (return to station) for a new gurney because the mattress was soaking wet. I told my partner we should keep the gurney because that's probably the cleanest it has been since it came out of the factory!

Tuesday, 9-30-14, 9:22 p.m.

There are two more "oops" I decided to add. I'm sure you have heard the question "Do you want the good news or the bad news first?" We have all heard that. So, do you want the good oops or the bad oops first? I would rather end on a good note than a bad one, so I will tell the bad story first.

This is an incident I will never forget. Paramedics, like everyone else, are not perfect. Sometimes things just happen because of our imperfect natures. I am talking about accidents. At work, we sometimes have accidents that are the paramedic's fault and others that just happen (or are someone else's fault).

One night, about ten or so years ago, I was driving south on I-95 just north of the Rancho exit. We were in the middle lane and we needed to exit at Rancho to go to the post to which we were just assigned. I checked my side-view mirrors and put on my blinkers. I didn't see any cars, but there was a small black car in my blind spot. It had been raining earlier, so the road was still a little wet. I just barely bumped him and he spun around and hit the inside jersey wall. The ambulance did a ninety-degree turn and was going sideways down the freeway. One of my infrequent four-letter words slipped out. Can you blame me? I knew a little bit about emergency driving, so I kept my foot off the brake and turned the steering wheel toward the direction we were sliding. Phew! Made it safely to the outside emergency lane.

Unbeknownst to me, and to my dismay, a highway patrol car was somewhere behind me and saw the whole thing. Crap! He pulled over and got in the ambulance to talk to us. He was very professional and didn't make me feel stupid. I was doing a good enough job of that myself!

I called my supervisor and he came out to meet us on the freeway. He was cool about it. He said, "Shit happens." It sure does!

The patrolman gave me a ticket for unsafe lane change. Oh, well. But I haven't had an accident since then. This has stayed in the back of my mind since then and has made me more careful about lane changes.

Now to the other "oops." I believe I got my first cell phone in 2000. It was one of those old ones: buttons on the outside, not a flip phone or slider, no texting, no camera, just a basic boring phone. I was at hospital N, just about ready to leave. When I went outside, I got a call from my sister in Washington State. "Are you all right?" I was confused at first until she said she heard screaming. Oh...I was standing in the ER when one of the patients was screaming. My sister was the victim of pocket dialing. Mystery solved.

CHAPTER NINE

SUICIDES, SUICIDE ATTEMPTS, HANGINGS, JUMPERS, AND HOMICIDES

4-4-03, 3:00 a.m.
In February, my partner and I transported a sixty-year-old man who committed suicide by injecting himself with ground up castor beans mixed in acetone. The bean contains a substance call ricin, classified as a weapon of mass destruction. What a ruckus this caused. Hospital C and hospital B were shut down for several hours. My partner and I had to go to hospital C for a decontamination shower. The patient died at the hospital.

Friday, 5-30-03, 4:24 a.m.
Worked another eight-hour overtime shift last night. Were we slow or what! Our first call was a fifty-year-old woman who called her doctor and told him she was going to kill herself. Of course, he called Metro and we showed up. She was rude, called us names, and needed a severe attitude adjustment. On scene, I asked her why she wanted to kill herself. Said she had a stroke (one to two years ago), lost her job as a nurse, staying home all day, could never be as smart as us. She was walking and talking without any visible deficits. I felt like telling her she has a lot to be grateful for. Some people, after a CVA [cerebrovascular accident], have such severe deficits that they can't walk, talk, swallow…sometimes they even die!

Tuesday, 6-17-03, 9:12 a.m.
Last night, we had a thirty-seven-year-old woman who got in an argument with her boyfriend. He…

Wednesday, 6-18-03
I fell asleep midsentence! To continue: He saw her swallow a bunch of pills from a bottle. Then she went in her room. When we got there, pills were spilled all over the floor, bottles broken…

Friday, 6-20-03, 4:26 a.m.
Guess I fell asleep, or went to sleep, midstream, again! To continue:

Patient was being pulled up off the floor by Metro. She had a couple pills stuck to her face, two capsules sitting in her left ear, and several pills stuck to her clothing. I left them all there. It was pathetically funny. Metro put her on a Legal 2000 [psych hold].

Saturday, 7-19-03, 2:40 a.m.
Last night, all four of our transports were men who had been drinking and we put on backboards. The first guy was diving, then doing flips from the third-floor balcony of his apartment into a five-foot-deep swimming pool. On the last flip, he landed on his feet (in the pool) and fractured his heel. Idiot! The second man was jumping from an eight-foot patio roof into a swimming pool. On his last attempt, the gutter gave way and he fell on his back. Had two lumbar compression fractures.

Sunday, 10-19-03, 12:15 a.m.
Several years ago, we ran a call for a young man who jumped off the Stratosphere. He worked at a grocery store in Utah, got a girl pregnant, stole money from the store, came to Las Vegas, and lost the money. In a state of emotional stupidity (he must have been emotionally unstable to begin with), he jumped. He hit a couple times before he landed on his back in some short shrubs near the valet area.

When we pulled up, FD was already there. As I was walking up, someone said something about getting a backboard. Are you kidding me??? It would be a miracle for someone to survive a fall of that distance. His right leg was fractured and his right foot was up near his head. His jacket had been pulled up, covering his head. I had someone pull his jacket down to expose his face. His eyes were open and had a film over them. There was no obvious bleeding anywhere. The body doesn't explode like a watermelon would.

We ran on another jumper near the MGM. He jumped from about four to six stories. He landed on his feet and his heels were split open in several places. The skin was pale/white, no blood. I think the blood shunted from the impact. He was dead.

Thursday, 2-3-05, 9:26 a.m.
Our last call this morning was for a dead body that a woman saw near the Paris hotel. Yeah, right, he was probably just drunk and passed out. Sure enough, when we got to the call, there was a body

lying facedown on the concrete outside next to the parking garage. As we walked up, you could see blood on the ground under his head. His legs looked a little deformed. FD rolled him over to get a better look. Oh, boy! His face was flattened! A little lump of flesh sunk in where his eyes should be. Lovely, lovely! Bad day for this guy! Probably a jumper. He looked more messed up than the guy who jumped from the Stratosphere several years ago.

Monday, 2-28-05, 12:10 p.m.

I need to put in more entries about work. So, here goes—not in order, because I don't remember the days they happened. Got a call for an eighteen-year-old man trying to hang himself. It was at a group home for kids with drug problems. When we got there, he was lying on the bedroom floor. He was awake, had an abrasion around his neck from the shoelaces he had tied together, put around his neck, and tried to hang himself with in the closet—four times! He said he passed out for a while.

Initially, someone (one of the kids—by kids I mean teenagers or young adults) came in and took the string off his neck. Then the person left and the patient did it again! Same scenario. After the third time, he went into the kitchen, grabbed a fork, went back to the bedroom, and hung himself again. Some kid came in, got him down, and forcefully had to restrain him on the floor.

While he was hanging, he had to bend his knees because the clothing rod wasn't high enough. So, you tried hanging yourself four times? Where were the staff people when this was going on? They were busy hiding the knives in the kitchen. What were you going to do with the fork? "Stab myself in the neck." This young man (probably weighed about two hundred pounds) was bipolar, had a history of multiple street-drug use, and just got out of a mental facility several days ago. Had been feeling suicidal since then.

I've had several calls involving hangings. Let's see: woman hung herself from the bathroom doorway—dead; man hung himself (or someone else did) from the railing on the street above the wash (Desert Inn and Mojave); woman who hung herself from the bathroom doorway in the upstairs bedroom. She had called her mother making suicidal threats. But instead of calling 911, the mother drove over there and arrived twenty minutes later. She was dead. FD was starting to work her, but she was asystole. I called the hospital, explained the situation, and the doctor said to stop resuscitation efforts.

I've had several calls that, fortunately for the patient, weren't successful. Silly young man tried to hang himself from a tree, but—duh!—didn't like the way it felt, couldn't breathe very well, and managed to swing his leg to a tree branch and stop the suicide attempt.

Suicide is very selfish. I remember a police officer friend said that one time. These people aren't thinking about others and how it may affect them. They also are usually blowing their situation way out of proportion. Killing yourself over a lost love, lost money, etc. Sometimes life really sucks and you have to suck it up! Of course, most people do. "Nothing in life is worth making yourself miserable over" (quote from Robert Fishman, PhD). "Nobody loves me, everybody hates me, think I'll eat some worms!"

Tuesday, 7-24-07, 12:27 a.m.

At work now—sitting in a parking lot at Silverado Ranch and Maryland Parkway. So far, we've run two calls in this general area. On the last call, one of the firemen said he was on the call of my accident. He said he'd never seen anyone so calm under those circumstances. He said they had trouble getting me over the jersey wall. I was on a backboard and my left leg slipped off the board. I calmly asked them to put it back. I don't remember that.

Last Thursday at about 2:30 a.m., we received a call for a man down. And he was down in the worst way! He was murdered! A tall, blond female was on scene. She said she just got out of jail and came back to her room (at a motel on Tropicana). A couple days ago, she met a man who she says was a rapper. Tonight, she walked in the room and he was lying facedown on the bed with a plastic grocery bag tied over his head. His hands were tied with a cord behind his back. She tore off the plastic bag and rolled him over. Then 911 was called.

The room was trashed. Suitcase, clothing, personal items, etc., were all over the floor. The bed headboard, initially secured to the wall, was hanging from the right corner. The man was lying supine, perpendicular on the bed. His right hand was under his lower back. I walked in first and put the monitor on the bed. The man looked dead, not breathing. My partner lifted up his left arm which was lying alongside his body. "He's rigored!" I did the same. He had been dead awhile. The female said she called him at about dinnertime while she was still in jail.

Realizing this was a crime scene, we didn't touch or move anything. The man had a thin layer of blood near his nose and there was blood smeared in the bag. While I was off work due to my injury (10-17-05), I watched a lot of *CSI Las Vegas*. I thought about *CSI* and looked at the man again. No ligature marks around his neck. Let's see. Any other obvious trauma? I didn't see anything. Metro showed up and we stayed for a few minutes until they cleared us.

Wednesday, 7-16-08, 8:31 a.m.
Yesterday (actually early this morning), we had a fifty-nine-year-old woman, weighed only 116 pounds, jumped (or was she pushed?) out of a two-story window onto the pavement below. She complained of neck pain, butt pain, and had a fractured right wrist. She said she jumped feet first and probably landed on her butt. When we got there, FD was holding manual C-spine and she was lying on her back. She was awake and talking. Except for the fractured right wrist, there were no other obvious injuries. Of course, she had been drinking, which contributed to that amazingly stupid event.

Tuesday, 6-2-09, 10:01 a.m.
Last night, we got a call for a self-inflicted gunshot. It was in a nice area near Buffalo and Washington. We didn't know what to expect. We were directed around to the backyard. Metro and FD were already there. The swimming pool was red tinged and in the middle was a man floating facedown just below the surface. FD got a long-handle pool broom and moved him over to the edge (after Metro took pictures). Then they pulled him out supine onto a backboard (board normally used to put accident patients on). He was thirties to early forties. GSW [gunshot wound] to the left side of his head with exit wound on the right. It was still dripping blood.

FD was being extra careful to check his pulses. About a month ago, a fire captain canceled the ambulance on a call for a guy who was shot. FD left the scene and the ambulance had driven around the corner to call their supervisor. Metro was on scene and called to have someone come back. The man was still breathing! Oops!

Tuesday, 7-5-11, 8:10 p.m.
I have been meaning to write about a call we had on June 1. We got

a call for someone who fell down a couple steps and was unresponsive. On the way to the call, I was thinking, "How could someone injure themselves so much from falling down a couple steps that they would become unresponsive?" When we got there, a young man was sitting on the couch downstairs. He told me he was having problems with his relationship with his "boyfriend." The boyfriend was upstairs while he was downstairs. While the patient was upstairs, he took too many of several different pills and chugged down some alcohol. And he cut his arms, neck, and upper legs numerous times. I asked him why he cut himself. He said he is a cutter and that is the only way he knows how to deal with emotional pain.

CHAPTER TEN

LIFE: THE SO-SO, BAD, AND UGLY

Monday, 5-12-03, 7:18 a.m.
Another "lovely" weekend. And because you can't hear the tone of my voice, the quotes are for denoting sarcasm! Late Saturday night, Brianna and I decided we were going to make chicken and rice. I bought a small chicken because it was on sale for $0.57/pound. It fit nicely into my favorite large stainless steel frying pan that can be used in the oven because the handle is metal, too. When the chicken was done, I took it out of the oven, using a pot holder, and set it on the stove. I was talking, distracted, and, not thinking, grabbed the handle to lift the pan without a pot holder. Aarrgh!!! And I think a four-letter word escaped, too! I rushed over to the sink to put my left (fortunately) hand under the cold water. For the next four hours I kept a ziplock sandwich baggie with water and a couple ice cubes in the palm of my hand. If I removed the baggie for more than fifteen to twenty seconds, it was very painful. I now have two burn marks diagonally across my palm. About half of it is blistered. I thought it would be a big problem last night at work. But I put several bandages on it, and fortunately, we had a slow (three transports), skinny patient (not over 170 pounds) night.

Wednesday, 4-7-04, 12:28 p.m.
Well, it's back to the point where I have to work overtime every weekend. Last pay period I worked three overtime shifts. This pay period only one. For the next one, I will have at least three. A one-income family just doesn't make it very easily. Yesterday, I added up all the bills I need to pay. It came to over $2,700 (that includes the mortgage). How depressing! I figured the only way out would be to cash out on some vacation time. So I called payroll yesterday and they said that I would have to get permission because I've already cashed out my maximum of ten shifts. So I filled out the request form and attached a note explaining why I needed it: car broke down, air-conditioning doesn't work, plumbing problems, and bills are killing me. They told me today (on the phone) that I'll get the check tomorrow. That sure took a load off. Unfortunately, though,

that leaves me only eight hours of vacation time.

Tuesday, 8-10-04, 2:13 a.m.

Yesterday, I didn't sleep after I got home. Evan and a couple friends went with Brianna to the airport to pick up Brianna's friend. Later, they all went over to another friend's house for a little while. I was watching the Yankees game. Tired, tired. The Yankees were disappointing me, so I decided to take a nap. Around 1:30 p.m., the kids got home and Evan came into my room. He knelt by my bed and said he had bad news. At first, I couldn't tell if he was kidding or serious. Then he spilled the "wonderful" news. He was hitting a punching bag and hurt his right wrist. There was some minor deformity on the outer radius. (About four to five years ago, he fractured his right wrist radius and ulna just superior to the growth plate.) I took him down to the doctor's office for an X-ray. Yup, he had a greenstick fracture of his radius. He got a brace to wear until his appointment at the orthopedic office—hopefully tomorrow (today). If his deformity were more obvious, then I would have taken him to hospital A.

Monday, 2-14-05, 6:56 a.m.

Saturday night, Braden was messing around and was trying to pick me up. I resisted and somehow slammed my chest real hard on his left shoulder. Man, that hurt! Now it hurts to breathe and move. I hugged a work friend from the other ambulance company and it hurt so much I let out a moan of pain and scared him. Oops, sorry!

Saturday, 2-25-06, 9:17 p.m.

Some really terrible things have happened in Las Vegas recently. Several weeks ago, a police officer responded to a domestic call. When he got to the door, he was shot and killed. Boy, was that a big news story! Contributions were made for his family. His funeral was a great big deal here in Las Vegas. About a week after his death, they had his funeral and broadcast it on TV. Denise watched it on TV from 9:00 a.m. until about 4:00 or 5:00 p.m. She had called me and told me she was glad I didn't die and she loved me. I was really touched by that. That afternoon, I went to a grocery store and bought three roses (shades of pink and red) made of feathers (quite beautiful; never seen feather roses before). I also got a vase. I already had a thank-you card at home, so I filled it out. About 1:00

or 2:00 p.m. I called her and asked if I could come over and show her something. Tyler drove me over. I went up to her door in the wheelchair. When she answered the door, I stood up and walked toward her. "Look, I can walk!" I said and gave her the flowers. She started crying and hugged me several times. She had already been real emotional from watching the funeral all day.

Monday, 4-17-06, 9:15 p.m.
Last Monday, I had an abdominal aortagram with runoffs. Basically, they shot contrast dye into my right femoral artery and traced its path through my descending leg arteries. When I had my appointment two days later with the doctor, they told me that the left leg artery just below the knee branches out into three vessels. The largest vessel is completely open. One other is completely occluded and one partially occluded. The open vessel has developed collateral circulation to the other two below the obstructions. What caused the obstructions? They didn't seem too sure, but I think they were trying to tell me they were from traumatic injury. The doctor said there was nothing they could do about them. There also is a problem with the veins. He said what I need is exercise, exercise—a lot of exercise—and in a couple years (!!!), I will probably be back to normal circulation. He reacted very positively to the news. But a couple years? I have been expecting to go back to work in a couple months!!! After the doctor left the exam room, my eyes started to well up with tears as I looked out the window. By the time I was getting in the elevator, tears were streaming down my face.

Comment: I have no doubt that the vascular damage was caused by my accident (Chapter 7). As of today, 3-27-12, my circulation is still not normal. And I don't think it ever will be. I have to wear compression knee-high stockings most of the time. And that really sucks during the summer when it's over one hundred degrees outside!

Tuesday, 5-2-06, 11:21 p.m.
Sunday night, Evan and a friend went to Walmart. I told all my kids I didn't want them going there alone, especially at night. Well, they said they were in the store for maybe only five minutes and when they came outside, the car was gone! Someone stole my car! I was upset, of course. But the tears didn't come until the next morning.

Man, I don't need this.

Sunday night, Brianna was really upset. It was my older station wagon that Brianna usually drives (to work, school, etc.) that was stolen. They don't drive my car (2004 Saturn Ion). Of course, they called Metro and filled out a report. The car was parked close to the front doors of Walmart and was (or should be) in plain view of one of the cameras.

Well, this morning I got a call that my car was located and I could pick it up at the tow yard. Why couldn't they just have called me when they found it? Metro did that once before when someone stole Tyler's truck. It cost me $141.70 to get my car out of the tow yard! Is Metro in cahoots with the towing companies? Tyler was even suggesting that the towing company towed it off, or took it, so they could generate revenue! I want to call Metro and ask them if they looked at the videotape, where they got the car, etc.

Comment: I really don't think Metro is in cahoots with the towing company or that the towing company stole it to generate revenue! Sometimes you say/write things you really don't mean when you're pissed off!

Wednesday, 6-7-06, 11:14 p.m.

Brianna and I were just discussing the possibility of publishing my journals. The whole topic came up after I had a hissy fit when I found the power bill sitting on the table by the couch. In Las Vegas, during the summer, that is one piece of mail I dread! $303.00! Why don't you just shoot me! I have to pay the mortgage and numerous other bills on Monday. And they'll probably be about twice the amount I get for workman's comp. I've been stressing about finances quite a bit lately. And the power bill was like the top of a pressure cooker blowing off. I yelled at Tyler to get a job and slammed my bedroom door behind me. I can't go to work!!! How am I going to get enough money to pay the bills? Yesterday, I canceled the cable movie channels. What more can I do?

Comment: Obviously, I forgot to look on the bright side. We had a place to live and we weren't starving! In fact, we were more fortunate than many people. But it is hard to think that way when you're stressed out.

Monday, 7-31-06, 6:31 p.m.
Yuck, I have to go to the DMV next week (or very soon) to renew my driver's license. Is there anyone in the world who likes to go to the Department of Motor Vehicles? If so, they need therapy!

Thursday, 9-21-06
Yesterday, my mother called me. She went in Tuesday to have cataract surgery on her right eye. She had it done on her left eye this summer and everything went fine. This time, something went wrong with the anesthesia and Mom stopped breathing. They called for an ambulance and Mom woke up in the ambulance. She was taken to the hospital. They did numerous tests, CAT scans, etc. Everything OK. I asked Mom to find out what kind of anesthesia was used, etc., and let me know. I am so thankful my mother is OK.

Comment: If I remember correctly, regarding the previous entry, the anesthesia (Lidocaine) traveled down the optic nerve to her brain stem and caused the respiratory arrest.

Tuesday, 10-17-06, 9:12 p.m.
One year ago today, I was lying in the trauma center with a mangled leg. I've been out of work for a whole year now. It's killing me, man! Most of my bills are late. And I didn't get my workman's comp check on Monday like I should have because the insurance company isn't on top of things. I have $2.34 in my checking account, after borrowing $100 from a cash advance place and $200 from a different one, so my water wouldn't be shut off, to buy a little bit of food, gas money, and a couple small bills (that go through automatically). Couldn't pay my mortgage yet. Late again for the second month in a row. I called the insurance company Monday. Check wasn't sent. They will FedEx it Tuesday morning. Called this afternoon and it still wasn't sent. So they set up the FedEx check while I was on the phone. But I won't get it until Thursday or Friday. I have to pay my power bill!

Friday, 10-27-06, 10:03 p.m.
My financial situation just keeps getting worse. I NEED to go back to work!!!!! I've had to adopt the attitude "Oh, well!" Only the absolutely essential bills are being paid, like power, water, mortgage...Any medical bills, credit cards, whatever, I'm trying to

ignore.

Wednesday, 1-10-07, 9:39 p.m.
Comment: This entry was written about a couple things that happened in the hospital after my accident on 10-17-05.

I don't think I ever wrote an account of my lung problems in the hospital or the problems with my toes. So, of course, by now the exact dates may not be exact.

Lung problem: On about 11-1-05, had video-assisted thoracoscopic surgery evacuation of a left hemothorax. That was on Tuesday. About the previous Tuesday or Wednesday (October 25 or 26), I was feeling a little short of breath, my chest felt a little tight, and I felt a little pain when I touched my left chest. I kept my cool, but I was getting very concerned. Was it my heart? I told the nurse and, being a paramedic, told her I wanted my pulse ox checked, a 12-lead, and a chest X-ray. I'm normally not bossy, but this was important. My pulse ox was 85 percent on room air. Bit too low for me, or anyone! The 12-lead EKG was normal. But the chest X-ray showed I had a problem. I had a hemothorax!

A chest tube was placed while I was *awake* in my room. Some pain meds were used, but WOW, that hurt! Twenty-five hundred cc of blood was drained!

The next day, I had an X-ray that showed blood/blood clots weren't all coming out. A bigger chest tube was put in. This time, he had trouble getting the proper placement. He kept moving it around. You're torturing me, man! Someone else was called to finish the placement.

Next day, X-ray wasn't good either. This time, the lung surgeon placed another tube, leaving the other one in. There were tubes from my chest to the collection receptacle (don't know what it's called). That first day, there sure was a lot of blood. Actually, I was surprised I wasn't more short of breath. Unfortunately, the three chest tubes didn't do the trick. So I went to surgery on Tuesday.

OK, now the toes. Had toe problem before lung problem. On 11-7-05, Kim (my sister) wrote "toes looking better." I remember my left toes started hurting and became bluish. I remember one night the pain was so intense the only thing that would relieve it was when Kim put my toes between her hands and squeezed. She would hold it for a while and after she released it I was OK for maybe twenty minutes. Then the pain came back. ALL NIGHT LONG! Kim actually set her alarm (she slept at my bedside for about a month!) to get up several times to help me. So my therapy (after that night) was to move my toes frequently to improve the circulation. Oh, well! Ended up with hard black necrotic tissue (dry gangrene) on my left big toe and second toe. The consensus of the doctors was to let nature take its course. May lose a toe or part of one.

Comment: The problem with my toes was caused by small blood clots that traveled to my toes. Eventually, I did lose about half inch of my left big toe and half of my second toe. The second toe is a nub and doesn't have a toenail. So, if I get a pedicure, would I get a 10 percent discount?

Thursday, 3-29-07, 12:56 p.m.
Several days ago, in the afternoon (I think), Brianna and I were standing in the kitchen. Suddenly, Brianna said, "Mom, there's a black man in our backyard!" I looked toward the dining room sliding glass door and saw a young black man walking by toward the corner of the house. (Thursday, 4-5-07, 3:37 p.m.) I quickly hobbled into the living room and asked Tyler to see why that man was in the backyard. I wasn't going to approach him because I'm still having trouble walking.

Tyler said later that he found him huddled by the outside chimney. Tyler had questioned him and the guy actually had the gall to try to go back into our backyard. Tyler held out his arm to stop him. Just then, he (Tyler) saw a police officer out front. Guess the black man noticed the look on Tyler's face and turned and started to run. Tyler ran after him, barefoot, through the rocks, only able to grab his T-shirt momentarily. Tyler fell partially in the grass, while the man slipped on the driveway in front of my car. He took off, but was apprehended by the officers (school police, I think—the patrol car was dark—not Metro) at the corner of the cul-de-sac. Boy, do I need to get gates put back up at the sides of my house! Last year, someone came into the backyard and stole our ladder.

Wednesday, 10-17-07, 10:26 a.m.
Last night (actually this morning at 1:25 a.m.), Brianna sent me a text message: "It's officially been two years since your accident, and I just wanted to say I love you and I'm thankful you're here :-)

XOXO." When I first read it, I was touched and I read it to my partner. But later, as we were sitting at the Tropicana and Fort Apache post, parked in a back parking lot where you can see the cars go by on I-215, I read it again. It really hit me then, and tears rolled down my cheeks. My partner was talking on her cell phone to one of her male friends, so I turned my head and looked out the window.

Friday, 10-19-07, 5:20 p.m.
I survived my second anniversary of my accident. Wednesday, at about 8:00 p.m., it was two years. Boy, was it an emotional night. Our first call was a Code 2 [non-urgent] transfer of an elderly man with anemia from hospital F to rehab. Before we went to the patient's room at hospital F, my partner needed to use the restroom. I stood in the hallway waiting for her and glanced at the room number of the rehab on my pager. Oh, no! Room 300! That was *my* room number! That room was different than most of them. The door off the main hallway led into a mostly empty room with a bathroom on the left end. Room 300 was next to the bathroom.

As soon as we entered the entrance room with the gurney, a rush of memories overcame me. The tears welled up in my eyes and I lost it! So many strong, painful memories—not just physical pain. The next hour, I struggled to compose myself. What irony! On the anniversary of my accident I end up transporting someone to the same room I stayed in for about a month!

7-3-09
I mentioned earlier that I have been having chest pains and a mild cough since February. I finally got a chest X-ray (in late May) and the report said: "AP [anterior-posterior] diameter of chest is increased with pulmonary hyperaeration consistent with emphysema. No evidence of pulmonary disease." How did I get emphysema? I've never smoked, not much exposure to environmental substances, no childhood diseases…

Comment: Not long after July 2009, something occurred to me. I have been using aerosol hair spray for YEARS! I'm sure that wasn't good for my lungs. So I stopped using aerosol hair spray and my chest pain soon diminished. I still get chest pain off and on, along with coughing. I wished someone would have slapped me on the side of my face years ago and said, "Stop that! You're damaging your lungs!" But isn't life sometimes like that? "Wish I hadn't done that" events!

Tuesday, 2-9-10, 6:37 a.m.
This is one journal entry that I truly wish I didn't have to write. But life has its joys and sorrows and sometimes (often) we have no control over them.

Last Saturday (February 6), Tyler and I went to Walmart and were planning on going to the store a little later. The Super Bowl was Sunday and he wanted to have a little party, have a friend over, and make some hamburgers and hotdogs. He also wanted me to make some chocolate cupcakes with cream cheese frosting. He had an idea. If you put some of the frosting in little ice cube trays and freeze it, then you could put a little piece in the middle of the cupcakes and have a creamy middle. He took some of the recipe books out of the cupboard and was going to try to find a recipe for that.

Ava's other grandmother was coming over around 3:30 to pick up Ava so they could spend the weekend together. After she picked up Ava, I decided to take a nap. Sometime around 6:00 p.m., Tyler came and woke me up and asked me if I would take him to 7–Eleven to get some beer. His chest had been bothering him for about forty-five minutes. He thought it was the discomfort from his occasional episodes of atrial fibrillation (irregular heartbeat).

I took him down to his usual 7–Eleven, parked along the side, and watched as he went in. The thought crossed my mind: "What if he collapses in there?" Then he came out and I drove us home. The receipt I later found had purchase time of his beer and pack of cigarettes at 6:12 p.m.

He went into the kitchen and bent over, leaning on the counter. I told him to take a beer and go sit down and I would put the others in the fridge. I felt his pulse a couple times and was a little surprised that it was regular. He wasn't in a-fib [atrial fibrillation]. He said, "I can't believe you can't feel it." He took a couple gulps of beer and said he just needed to relax. But he couldn't.

This was the worst chest pain he has ever had. He said it was squeezing, with pain up into his neck and in his left arm. He felt short of breath and he was starting to sweat. I told him we needed to call 911. He didn't want to because then he would have to go to the hospital. Finally, he said, "You better call." So I called. Then he said, "I didn't want to go this way. I wanted to die in my sleep."

Knowing I was going to go with him, I went to my room to get my coat (it was raining) and use the bathroom. I was gone for only a minute or less. When I got back to the living room, Tyler had gone into cardiac arrest while sitting on the couch. Before my stupid, unfortunate trip to the bathroom Tyler had told me that he was feeling short of breath even when he was scrubbing the pans lately. Why didn't he tell me?

I have been suffering over this—why did I leave him for that minute? Why did I let him die by himself on the couch? Why didn't I stay by his side and comfort him? I know the outcome would not have changed, but I should have showed more compassion. How could I? I sat in my closet on the floor last night, crying, torturing myself about my stupidity and insensitive act…Then I decided I couldn't keep doing this. It wasn't healthy or productive and I don't think Tyler would want me to do that.

So after I got back to the living room and was totally shocked at what had happened (I was imagining in my mind that he would go to the hospital, of course get the cardiac workup in the ambulance, and then probably have surgery), I said, "Help me get him down on the floor." Now I don't remember who helped me, probably Evan.

I started chest compressions and did some mouth-to-mouth ventilations. I told Brianna to call 911 back and tell them he was in cardiac arrest. Tyler still had some agonal respirations.

The fire department arrived first and put the patches on his chest. He was in v-fib. Their stupid monitor malfunctioned and wouldn't shock. So there was a few minutes delay until the ambulance arrived.

I did chest compressions the whole time they were working on him. He was intubated, an IV started, and received some drugs. I really wanted him to be transported to hospital B, but the fire medic said—and I knew it was true—hospital F is closer, so we have to go there.

I rode in the front of the ambulance. The driver was kind of new, was driving a little slower that I would have, but he was trying to give his crew a smooth ride. And it was raining. I wanted to say, "Can't you drive a little faster?" but I knew the hospital wouldn't do anything much different than what they were doing. On the way to the hospital, I called my mom and asked her to say a prayer for Tyler. Of course, I was already praying. But I think I did mention

"Thy will be done." I wasn't expecting any miracles.

After some of the shocks, his rhythm changed to PEA [pulseless electrical activity] and then went back into v-fib. They worked him for ten to fifteen minutes at the hospital. Sometime during that, I called home to let the kids know what was going on and asked if Evan could give me the phone number of some friends from church. I wanted someone with me at this time who knew, like I know (faith), that this life is not the end. I wanted some spiritual comfort.

We waited at the hospital until 10:30 p.m. for the coroner. Tyler was pronounced at 7:19 p.m. Because of the rain, the coroner's office was busy with traffic fatalities. The hospital had me sign a paper, they gave me the info on the funeral home, and my friends took me home.

What a miserable night! My poor kids! They had some issues with their father, but they still loved him. Tyler's father died at the same age—fifty-four. His father was outside in the backyard, walked into the kitchen, and collapsed on the floor.

Friday, 12-24-10, 2:00 p.m.
Thursday morning, I had a scary, almost disastrous, incident. Work was over and I was just headed home. I was sitting at the red light at Charleston and MLK, headed east to get on the freeway. Don't know what really happened. It felt like I had a few seconds when my brain went blank. All of a sudden I heard a car honking and I was in the middle of the intersection going against the red light. I saw a car coming at me and I swerved to the right, just missing it (car was turning left, going south). Holy crap!!! What did I do? Was I day dreaming, saw the green arrow, and went without thinking? I don't remember even noticing the light. Did I fall asleep at the intersection? Freaked me out! Both Tuesday and Wednesday I didn't get much sleep (three and a half to four hours).

Wednesday, 2-9-11, 8:03 a.m.
This last Sunday, February 6, was the Super Bowl. I didn't watch any of it. Didn't care. Kind of a rough weekend for us, especially me and Brianna. February 6 last year was when Tyler died. It was the day before the Super Bowl.

Saturday, something kind of bizarre happened. Ava and I were sitting at the kitchen counter eating breakfast. Out of the blue, she asked, "Where's Grandpa?" I asked her if she knew what happened to him. She said, "He died." Then she asked, "Who killed Grandpa?" I explained to her that his heart was sick and that sometimes when people are too sick, they die. She also asked about the dog (Paris). He died (11-30-09) before Grandpa did.

Sunday, 2-27-11, 3:28 p.m.
It's still the same old, same old thing—working twelve-hour shifts, missing sleep especially on Wednesday to Friday to watch Ava in the morning after I get home from work. On my first day off, I'm tired all day. I remember once, a couple years ago, waking up and feeling good and refreshed. Wouldn't that be nice!

Comment: That previous entry is a pretty pitiful statement! But I still don't wake up refreshed. My neck is sore and feels stiff, and I can feel a headache coming on. I started taking generic Excedrin a while back to help with the neck pain and occasional headache. Then I started taking it at work once in a while to help me get through the night. Can't work safely when you're too tired. Now I take a pill every morning and usually in the late afternoon. It sucks getting "hooked" on caffeine! But nothing else helped me with my headaches. Complain, complain, complain…Look on the bright side! It's better than being hooked on heroin, pain meds, cigarettes.

Sunday, 4-17-11, 7:28 p.m.
A week ago Friday, at about 3:00 a.m., while I was at work, I got a call from Braden. He has a part-time job now delivering newspapers. He uses my truck and had a tire blow out on the freeway, southbound 95 just before the Flamingo exit. We had been really slow at work (our first transport was after midnight—shift starts at 5:45 p.m.). I called the sup and asked if we could rescue my son. Ava's father was with him. So we picked them up (in the ambulance) and drove to my house. Braden used Brianna's car to do his route. First had to get the papers out of the truck. After I had dropped them off at the house, we went back to work. I had ordered a spare for the truck the weekend before because the truck didn't have one. Good thing I did!

The next morning, Braden and I picked up the spare and went out to the freeway. Had to jump-start the truck, too. While he was changing the tire (it was the rear driver's side) I kept thinking, "God, please don't let anyone hit us!" We survived our little adventure. I've heard terrible stories of what happens to people stranded on the freeway!

Comment: What freaked me out most about changing a tire on the freeway was the terrible uneasiness I felt because of my accident on the freeway. It takes a long, long time to get over something like that! I felt very uneasy just walking on the sidewalk for a long time.

Sunday, 6-12-11, 2:44 p.m. (actual day of occurrence 6-4-11, after returning home from a meeting)

After I got home (about 3:30), Ava told me she threw up. Poor thing! Brianna said she threw up about five times. She has been coughing for a few days. So I'm not sure if she threw up because she has been coughing so hard or not.

Shortly after I got home, Ava was lying down on my bed and I noticed she was breathing fast. I counted her respirations and it was at about eighty times a minute. And she was using her abdominal muscles. Pulled out my trusty stethoscope and she was wheezing a little with slightly diminished tital volume in her lower lung fields.

I had told Erin that if Ava doesn't get better I was going to take her to quick care in the morning. Different story now. Evan came with me to take her to the hospital. Ava was so upset. She wanted to take a nap.

As we were driving down Bonanza, Ava was crying and pointing behind her, "I want to go back there!" She kept saying it over and over. She wanted to go back to the house. Of course I knew better. We went to hospital C peds.

They took her right back to a room. With oxygen sats of 92 percent, an elevated respiratory rate, wheezes, and accessory respiratory muscle use, you do get a bed right away! She was given some oral Decadron and put on an SVN [small-volume nebulizer] Albuterol for an hour. She handled that mask so well! What a trooper!

Before she had the treatment (or was it after?), Ava was talking a lot with the nurse and doctors. One doctor came up to her and she started asking questions. "Have you seen *Tangled*?" Once when the nurse was standing nearby, Ava looked at Evan and said, "You're a butt munch!" Made the nurse laugh.

She started to run a fever (101), so they gave her some

Tylenol. At first, the doctor was calling it reactive airway disease. That's what they call the early stages of asthma for children. Later, I talked with her other grandma and she said Ava's father has asthma. Great! Chances are good that Ava may get asthma, too! That sucks!

CHAPTER ELEVEN

MISCELLANEOUS MEDICAL PROBLEMS

5-2-03, 4:47 a.m.
The next call was for a man with a history of alcoholism. He lives with his mother. She said he had a seizure at 5:00 p.m., then one this morning. He was a bit postictal when we got there, but he was coming around and refused to go to the hospital. FD was filling out the AMA (against medical advice) form.

I asked the patient to sit down again because I wanted to put him on the monitor. His head was soaked with sweat. Before I could get the leads on, he went into another seizure for about one and a half minutes. Later, my partner told me she could see his toes starting to curl under just before his body started shaking. Before he came around, we put him on the gurney and then took him out to the ambulance. I told someone in the break room while I was writing the report that he probably was seizing because his alcohol dip stick was low.

Saturday, 9-6-03, 11:05 p.m.
Last night, I worked a twelve-hour overtime shift. For now, they won't let us work eight-hour overtime. They want the regular twelve-hour shifts filled first. We got a call at Vegas and Rancho for a 32B (unknown problem) man complaining of feeling like he's going to pass out, at pay phone at a 7–Eleven, wearing a green shirt. En route, I said to my partner, "It better not be Fred [name changed]!"

As we pulled up, there was a man in a green shirt, walking with his back to us, smoking. We honked the air horn at him and he turned around. As I walked up to him, I realized it was Fred. Probably our current worst 911 abuser. (I feel the frustration churning inside of me. I'm chomping on crackers, peanuts, and drinking diet cola while writing this…and listening to Cher.) He's an alcoholic. Calls 911, gets transported to the hospital, walks out shortly afterward, walks a short distance, and then calls 911 again, etc., etc.

My partner said she transported him three times in one day. I transported him for the first time last week to hospital B. He supposedly couldn't walk—too drunk. We put him in triage at the hospital. As we were pulling away from the hospital, we saw him walk out the door, walking just fine.

Tuesday, we took him back to hospital B. He was more intoxicated. As we were waiting for a bed, I heard the sound of fluid dripping on the floor. Fred was passed out on our gurney, started urinating, and it ran down to the foot of the gurney and dripped onto the floor. Nearby, a nice-looking man was lying on a gurney watching it all. I made a few faces off and on and he saw it. I ended up talking to him, discussing how we feel about bringing drunks to the hospital versus patients like him. He had a back injury. He made a comment about seeing me before while I was working out on the street (probably at an accident). I said, "We get around!"

Wednesday, 10-1-03, 6:56 a.m.
Last night, I had one of those calls when I feel like a jerk for ever complaining about my life. We got a call for a forty-one-year-old male with terminal cancer. His girlfriend called because he seemed to be hallucinating. Metro responded and while they were there, he had a short seizure and stopped breathing. Then we got notes en route that he coded. Immediately, we wondered if he has DNR (do not resuscitate) papers.

When we got there, we found he was breathing again. One of the officers there used to work for us. The patient was lying on his bed with his girlfriend kneeling beside him. We talked with him for a short time and then asked if he had DNR papers. The girlfriend said, "DNRs?" and started crying very emotionally. Obviously, she knew what they are and he hadn't told her.

His doctor had the DNRs. We told him if he codes, we have to work him if he doesn't have the form in his apartment. He's going to get it today. He has only two months to live. That really sucks! Forty-one years old and to have death staring you in the face.

Wednesday, 10-15-03, 10:59 (in reference to 10-14-03)
Several hours after that, we had a call at the 7–Eleven on Eastern and Sahara. It was a deaf man who was put out of his apartment four days ago. He had two grocery carts full of belongings. He

complained of pain in his shunt (head) and dizziness. What he really wanted was a place to go. We spent more than one hour writing notes back and forth on little 7–Eleven paper bags that I opened up. We told him we could take him to the hospital, but we couldn't take all of his stuff.

At one point, he took a knife out of his pocket and held it to his neck. He was pretty calm the whole time. Think he was trying to show us his state of desperation. I wrote asking if he could call his social worker later in the morning. My partner laughed at me—he's deaf. The patient laughed a little. I wrote, "Sorry. Duh! Brain fart." He wrote "Stop, silly." A little levity toward him and he took me by the arm for a second in a suggestive friendship gesture.

Metro pulled up. Guess he saw us and stopped to see if we were OK. The officer ended up loading all of the patient's belongings into his trunk and backseat and gave the patient a ride to St. Vincent's (a shelter). It was 2:00 a.m., so they probably weren't accepting anyone, but he could hang outside until they opened. Nice police officer! Not all of them are that helpful.

Thursday, 10-16-03, 7:31 a.m.
Thought last night was going to be boring. Toward the beginning of the shift, we were sent to Silverado Ranch and Las Vegas Boulevard. We sat there at the gas station for probably an hour. Then I heard sirens and saw Metro going south on I-15 and stop. Then another Metro went south on Las Vegas Boulevard, turned around, and went north (guess he was trying to get over to I-15). Then we got the call. Nevada Highway Patrol (NHP) and Metro had I-15 southbound, just south of Blue Diamond, blocked off. There was a little confusion on where our patient was, so I stopped and NHP came over to talk with us. A Metro car nearby shined his spotlight at us. I thought, "What is this doofus doing?" NHP said our patient was up ahead. A pregnant lady. Well, the Metro "doofus" was someone I know. He was trying to get my attention.

I'm tired, more later.

(Same day, 3:30 p.m.) Our patient was a fifteen-year-old female, five months pregnant. She was with a male friend (young, mentally unstable) of hers and they went over to her (or his?) grandparents' house. He pulled a gun on them, made a suicidal threat, and told them he was taking her as a hostage. He forced his pregnant friend into his car and sped away from Pahrump toward

Las Vegas going speeds up to 100 mph. At one time, he hit a bump and she (not wearing her seat belt) flew up, hit her shoulder on the car roof, and came down hard on her rear end. She was complaining of abdominal pain. As we were talking with her outside (on the side of I-15), she started getting dizzy, so we went in the ambulance.

Thursday, 4-22-04, 11:10 a.m.

Our first patient last night was a "real winner"! Female in her seventies complaining of chest pain. On scene, to start off, she complained FD was talking too much. They were only asking the usual questions. She only liked me. I wasn't talking too much. Well, duh, I was listening to FD because they were there first. When we got back in the ambulance, my partner asked her some questions (I think about smoking). For some reason, she got really upset, started yelling and shaking her arms at him. After she calmed down a little, I told her he would be driving. She said, "Get up there and put some tape on your mouth!"

En route, while on the freeway, she wanted us to stop, let her out, and she would walk home. I wrote a note to my partner not to talk to her, don't worry about it, I'll call the supervisor to warn him in case she calls to complain. She wanted my partner's name, but I refused to give it to her.

Saturday, 5-8-04, 11:58 a.m.

Thursday night, we had a fifty-one-year-old female who, according to her male friend who just got out of prison, had been passing out numerous times in the past three days. She was also running into the walls, seeming a little confused, not eating, only drinking a lot of regular cola.

When we got there, she was lying on some blankets on the floor, wedged between the bed and nightstand. She was very lethargic, very weak, but alert. We lifted her (she weighed only about 120 pounds) onto the bed. Could not feel radial pulses. My partner could not get a blood pressure. I asked FD if they would get their auto BP cuff (it's part of the monitor). Her blood pressure was 53/28—probably one of the lowest BPs I've seen.

We got her down to the truck. I tried a left AC IV. It didn't work. FD got an IV in her left external jugular vein (neck). By the time we got her to the hospital, she received 575 cc normal saline. It only brought her BP up a little (60/30). We took her to hospital B.

Later, another crew brought someone with a low BP. A nurse told them Lynn's patient's BP was lower! No, it's not a contest. We checked her later and they had her in a pretty extreme Trendelenberg and her pressure was still real low. The nurse said she was acidotic and she was probably in renal failure. The kidneys help control blood pressure. I think this girl is really screwed up.

Tuesday, 7-27-04

Friday morning we stayed almost three hours overtime. We already got gas, were Code 86 (going back to the station), when we heard numerous trucks being called to an MCI (mass casualty incident) down south. We also were called. It was on Greer (off Sunset, east of Bermuda). People in some kind of communications building smelled an odor some described as a pesticide.

Everyone was evacuated and twenty-four people were transported. Some of the symptoms were nausea and vomiting. My patient, a young lady with asthma, had chest pressure, dizziness, and disorientation. At the time, the fire department couldn't find the cause.

We took our patient to hospital E. They made her decon— take off everything and take a shower. They gave me a choice. No way, baby! We didn't go in the hospital. Someone came out and took our report. While I was sitting outside on the cement, leaning up against a wall in the ambulance driveway writing my report, the CCT (critical care transport) ambulance drove up. He rolled down his window and commenced to order hamburgers, fries, etc. I got up, walked over to him, and asked if he wanted to biggie size that.

Monday, 8-23-04, 12:36 p.m.

This past week, I got off late every day. I took Friday (my birthday) off and worked OT on Saturday. Our last call came at 9:08 a.m. Per our pagers: "Patient violent, hasn't taken insulin for twelve hours." En route, I'm thinking, "He can't be violent because of his blood sugar. It wouldn't be low."

The patient lives in a group home for brain-injured people. Back in 1988, our patient went into a diabetic coma and suffered brain damage. He has episodes of violence. This morning was one of those. He refused to take the last two doses of his meds (for diabetes and seizures, including Ativan).

When we got there, the patient was in his bedroom, sitting on a couch. My partner opened the bedroom door, did not go in, and asked him if we could check his blood sugar. The patient yelled back, "I don't give a #%#& what you do!" Then he jumped up, grabbed something, and charged at the door. My partner quickly slammed the door shut and the patient pounded on the door, yelling. OK, we'll wait for Metro!

Metro struggled a little with the patient to get him on the floor and then handcuffed him. Then they stood him up so he could be put on the gurney. The patient kicked at one of the officers (a short, muscular, macho-looking guy). The officer said, "You kicked me in the balls!" I'm not sure he really connected. The officer lost it. I saw him swing at the patient with his fist. Later found out he hit him in the lateral left eyebrow area. (I couldn't see everything because I was standing outside the door.) There was a minor laceration just below the outer eyebrow.

On the way to the hospital, my partner was in the back and Metro was following us. Of course the patient was in four-point restraints. On the freeway, my partner yells at me, "He's having a seizure!" So I pulled over, turned on the lights, and went in back. I started an IV and we soon discovered, after the patient tried to fiddle in his pocket, that he had four (yes, four!) pocket knives in his pants pockets. What is a patient with a mental problem and a history of violence doing with knives! At the hospital, my partner filled out an incident report for Metro.

Comment: Usually, Metro will check a violent, or potentially violent, person for weapons. I guess they forgot! Sometimes, I ask Metro if they searched the person. I have never had anyone pull a weapon on me, but I have heard stories!

Sunday, 1-16-05, 4:22 p.m.
One week with my new partner. I like her. She's a good EMTI. We have a lot in common (divorced, kids...). She brought me dinner on Wednesday (teriyaki rice and noodles).

We've had a lot of critical patients lately. It was kind of peculiar. For four shifts in a row, the first patient was the most critical: altered mental status (maybe CVA [cerebrovascular accident]), an IC [intracerebral] bleed, a really severe stroke, and an MI ([myocardial infarction] heart attack) with tombstone elevation. The severe CVA was a woman in her fifties who fell at work and was found on the floor under a clothing rack. Her left side was totally flaccid. She had left facial droop, but fortunately was alert and able to talk. It was a little hard for her to speak when the left side of her mouth wouldn't move. And her head was cocked over to the right.

The IC bleed, which we took to hospital B, probably won't (or didn't?) have a good outcome. They think the bleed was in the lower back of her head (don't remember what they called it). The day we had the tombstone MI we also had another MI.

Thursday, 2-3-05, 9:26 a.m.
We had a middle-aged woman with a history of seizures and a brain tumor. Her boyfriend said she had six seizures in twenty minutes. Between each seizure he gave her a 1 mg Ativan by mouth. When we got there, she was pretty alert. By the time we got to the hospital she was "snowed"! Now we had an ingestional error, too! Five to six Ativans!

Tuesday, 6-7-05, 9:37 a.m.
We had a sixty-nine-year-old female who woke from sleep thirty minutes before our arrival (so about 1:30 a.m.) complaining of a severe headache. Five minutes before we got there, she passed out on the toilet. She had been vomiting also. My partner went up to her and felt her pulse. A code? No, she had good pulses, but she was breathing only three to four times a minute. Oh, I bet she had a bleed. We put her on a non-rebreather at 15 liters. We lifted her onto the gurney and took her out to the truck. I got her intubated.

We went back Code 3 [life threatening] to hospital N. The charge nurse made a comment that every time I go there I bring a critical patient. He said I should put CCT (critical care transport) on the side of my truck. Maybe so.

Recently, we took in a forty-nine-year-old man who went from "Ugh, something's going on, maybe" to tombstones (nickname for bad cardiac rhythm), at his house, in five minutes! Holy crap! Let's get going! I remember asking him, "Is your chest pain getting worse?"

Well, the lady from last night ended up with a severe intracranial bleed. The CCT transported her to hospital B (neurosurgeon on call).

We also had an eighty-year-old man who fell in the bathroom, coded, and by the time we got there, it had already been about twenty minutes. I don't think the family understood the urgency of his situation. Unfortunately, he was in asystole. How could he be otherwise after twenty minutes of no CPR?

Thursday, 7-24-08, 1:48 p.m.
Last night, we transported a young (twenty-four-year-old) woman to hospital G for a Legal 2000 [psych hold]. She was wacky! She wanted to be transported on the top of the ambulance. And en route, she told my partner she was born with a mohawk. "Just ask my dad." She said some other weird stuff, too.

She was incarcerated for two days on domestic violence. They said she liked to take her clothes off and get naked. Initially when the police picked her up, she was intoxicated. But after two days, she wasn't under the influence of anything except her psychotic mind.

Friday, 6-20-03, 4:26 a.m.
This a.m. we had a Code 2 [non-urgent] for a sixty-one-year-old lady with a bad rash. The call was at an urgent care. They were transferring her to hospital A. We thought, "Oh, brother! They can't take care of a rash?" When we got there, it was shocking! She had big red blotches all over her body (even on the palms of her hands). She had been taking ibuprofen and Darvocet every day for a month for knee pain. They think maybe it was the ibuprofen. She started breaking out on Monday and this was her third trip to a quick care. They had given her Prednisone, Benadryl, Solumedrol, Visteril...Her white blood cell count was 27.8 (thousand). The normal is about 4–10.

Comment: When I started reading this before I typed it, I let out a big "Ooh!" It was like a lightbulb suddenly turned on in my head. I wonder if she had the same thing I had in July 2010. I started breaking out in a rash a couple days after I had a CT [scan] with contrast done to check for the possibility of a PE [pulmonary embolism]. That day, I was seeing a dermatologist about a small lump (it was basal cell carcinoma) and showed him the rash. The rash got worse and the next week when I saw the doctor, he took a skin sample and had it sent off for a biopsy. It came back as leukocytoclastic vasculitis. The rash was all over my body, except for very little on my face. It took about two weeks for it to go away completely. I missed a couple days work because it was so itchy. So, no more CTs with contrast for me!

Sunday, 4-19-15, 10:58 p.m.
I just made brownies and put them in the oven. Don't bake goodies very often anymore. I eat too much of them. But once in a while, just gotta!

There are a few calls I would like to write about.

Last week, we got a call for a woman walking along Blue Diamond. This road heads out west toward Pahrump.

An off-duty Metro police officer saw her walking along the side of the road and called us.

When we got there, an elderly female and the officer were on the side of the road, several yards from traffic. She seemed to be keeping her distance from him. He said she wouldn't tell him much.

I walked up to her and we started talking. I liked her. She was a nice lady with a cute sense of humor.

She lives with her ex-husband and asked him in the morning (it was now about 1:30 p.m.) if he would drive her to Pahrump so she could visit her twin sister. He said it was too far. I guess that wasn't going to stop her. She left her home around sunrise, stopping somewhere to get a hamburger. She was holding a sixteen ounce bottle of water that was almost half empty.

After talking with her and Metro and NHP [Nevada Highway Patrol] for about twenty minutes and explaining, or trying to, that it wasn't a good idea for a seventy-year-old woman to walk to Pahrump, it suddenly occurred to me that we should check her vitals. Her blood pressure was OK, but her heart rate was 153! She had been standing there for at least twenty minutes, not exerting herself.

Metro decided to fill out a Legal 2000 if she wouldn't go voluntarily to the hospital. We managed to talk her into going to the hospital to get checked out.

She was able to answer all A & O [alert and oriented] questions appropriately, but her thinking process was not right. Probably has some dementia.

We transported her to hospital E, which was about twelve miles from where we picked her up. And add a couple more miles to her place. So she probably walked about fourteen or so miles.

She was a short lady and in pretty good shape. Said she walks where she wants to go. Doesn't drive or have a car.

The same day, I had my first near drowning.

A four-year-old boy was using some kind of floating device and there were other kids in the pool, including his older sister. His mother was nearby, but looked away momentarily. Then she saw him underneath the water. Imagine her panicked state! She quickly got him out and he wasn't breathing. She did CPR and water started coming out of his mouth. Then he started breathing.

FD said his sats were in the 80s. When we got there, he wasn't very responsive, but he was breathing. FD had him on an NRB [non rebreather].

I got an IV on him and we took him to hospital C peds. His lungs were clear.

Just before we got to the hospital, he was responding to me. I asked him if he hurt anywhere and he shook his head "no." Then I asked if he was having trouble breathing and he shook "yes."

The mother, of course, was upset and had a few tears, but she was keeping it together. We all told her she did a great job. And she did. Before I left, I gave her a hug and told her again that she did great.

CHAPTER TWELVE

ANIMALS

Comment: I decided to include a chapter on animals because…well…I have a lot of them, I love them, and they are my little friends. They are a part of my life.

Monday, 4-18-05, 3:05 a.m.

Brianna called me forty-five to sixty minutes ago. She and her boyfriend were driving down Betty, south of Lake Mead, and found a white cat lying in the road. Brianna said it was still breathing. They called 311 and I also gave them the number for animal control.

I drove over there (grabbed some gloves, stethoscope, and a box) to check out the condition of the cat. It was lying in the road, moving mostly its hind legs. It flopped over a couple times, tried to stand up, but couldn't. Looks like it got hit in the head. The lower jaw was broken and the tongue was hanging out. The skin around one eye was bloody and the other pupil was completely dilated. It had a nice strong heartbeat and wasn't in any respiratory distress. Brianna was crying.

I opened up the box and scooped the cat onto it and moved it next to the mailboxes. Brianna's boyfriend called again, gave the address, and they said they were on the way. Probably ten minutes later, the animal control truck showed up. The lady was very friendly. She pushed the cat into a cage and said she was taking it to an emergency hospital.

I told Brianna the cat probably has a serious head injury and they would have to put it down. Maybe it wasn't true, but I told her the cat may not be feeling any pain because of the head injury. So why did I pet the cat to try to comfort it? I hate seeing animals get hit by cars. Of course I'm not too crazy about people getting hit by cars. The animals are innocent creatures and don't know the dangers of "J walking." Why is it called J (or is it jay) walking?

Comment: I read over a few more journal entries (two kittens that died, how my three-legged cat lost his leg, etc.) and decided that I didn't want to include any more animal stories...except this next one. It's not depressing! Also, it happened at work. So it's part of being a paramedic!

Thursday, 9-11-09

We were on a call at an apartment complex. An eighteen-year-old female was at a party and drank a whole bottle of tequila. Her father went to pick her up and while trying to get her in the car, she became combative, hit her head, and got a nice shiner (black eye). Because she was not answering questions appropriately, she won a trip to the hospital.

My partner and I went to the back of the ambulance to get the gurney. I opened the back doors and, it seemed from out of nowhere, a large white dog ran up to the truck and tried to jump in the back. He got his front legs on the floor of the ambulance and I had to pull him off. My partner is afraid of dogs, so she did a quick about face. Then the dog tried to get in again. I pulled him out again and then he trotted over to a Metro patrol car and tried to get in.

Many years ago, I actually transported a lady with a seizure disorder who had a service dog to help her with her medical problem. I called the supervisor then and he said we could transport the lady with her dog as long as the dog was an official registered service animal.

CHAPTER THIRTEEN

TRAUMATIC INJURIES

Sunday, 9-14-03, 8:39 p.m.

Yesterday after ACLS [advanced cardiovascular life support] class, I went into one of the offices at work to ask about getting a new copy of the ACLS book. Suddenly, "HELLO!! HELLO!! HELLO!!" I went into the hall and saw an elderly gentleman with a panicky look on his face. He said there was a man, bloody, with his arm almost cut off. The person in the office called for FD and an ambulance.

I went outside with the man. He said the injured man was over on Wall Street. He walked over to a car parked crooked in the parking lot. He said he would give me a ride over. I told him I would go over and check him out. I thought for a couple seconds, "A stranger, elderly gentleman, genuinely distressed. Maybe I could help?" I accepted his offer and he drove us over to the site only two to three blocks away.

A young man was lying on the floor just inside the door of some kind of appliance warehouse. Down the hall, there were several refrigerators up against the wall. There was a belt wrapped around his left arm near the elbow, a towel over his forearm. I could see a straight laceration across the palm of his left hand. No bleeding. I asked them how long the belt had been on. Ten minutes. I asked them to take it off.

On the way over, I could see FD coming down the street. So they got there about thirty seconds after we did. When the fire crew walked up, I bit my tongue (not literally!) and said very little. A couple minutes later, the ambulance showed up. I knew the paramedic. He asked what I was doing there. Second job?

The bottom corner of a fridge had fallen on the man's arm. He had a three-to-four- inch laceration/evulsion on his forearm. There was only a slow bleed with minimal blood on scene. So, as FD pointed out, it wasn't an arterial bleed. They loaded the patient up and the same gentleman gave me a ride back to the station. He asked my name, introduced himself, and thanked me for coming over. I didn't do much, but mostly because FD and the ambulance arrived and I had to step back and let them do their job. Besides, I didn't have any gloves or equipment.

Sunday, 8-1-04, 2:20 p.m.

Tyler, Erin, and Brianna are in the living room watching some stupid show about rich, spoiled, newly married young stars. Make me puke! I'm sorry (not really), but rich, spoiled people irritate me! So I went into my bedroom and I'm watching *True Lies* with Arnold Schwarzenegger and Jamie Lee Curtis.

Friday morning, about 1:00 a.m., we ran a call for an auto-ped at Tropicana and Swenson. As we pulled up, FD had a man on a backboard. He appeared to have blood all over. "Oh, #!&#" was my first reaction. We have a serious patient! As I walked up, I saw a small stream of blood running from his neck area. It left a blood trail about six to eight feet long.

On the way to the trauma center, he was a real pain in the butt. He became combative, so we had to tie down his arms. Even then, he messed up two good IVs. His pupils were blown—7 mm. He had a fractured left tib/fib, a five-inch partial thickness laceration to the right side of his neck, and numerous small lacerations to his right forearm and elbow.

When we got to trauma, my partner warned them that the patient was combative. They didn't take him seriously at first, but they soon found out for themselves. He hit a doctor. He told them he had been doing "lots of drugs" (which may account for the dilated pupils). The CAT scan was not showing a head injury.

Before the accident, the patient was running across the street. The driver didn't see him and she hit him going 40–45 mph. The patient hit the windshield, leaving a big dent in the driver's side.

Saturday, 8-7-04, 12:22 p.m.

This morning we had a seventeen-year-old girl who got really depressed and cut herself numerous times on her forearms and upper legs with a razor. Her mother found her sitting on the bathroom floor. All the cuts were superficial and only a teeny bit of blood was visible. She was a lot calmer than would be expected.

Wednesday, 10-20-04, 11:38 a.m.

Some recent calls:

Sixty-two-year-old male went out into his garage to apparently sit and have a cup of coffee late at night. His daughter came out and found him. He had fallen out of the chair and slumped onto some stuff in front of the chair.

When she called 911, Metro was in the area, so they helped lay him down on the floor. When we got there, he was unresponsive and only breathing about eight times a minute. I thought, "Oh crap, this guy is going to code!" He had a history of three brain operations in the last year for hemorrhage. He had a shunt going down the back of his head, across his chest, and emptying (assumption) into his digestive system somewhere. You could see it underneath his skin on his right chest.

He started talking in the ambulance, but was confused. En route, he found the finger hole in the cabinet window and was moving it back and forth and saying "40, 45, 50." We first were en route to hospital D, but as I was talking to the charge nurse on the radio, she said that if we believe it could be another bleed problem we should divert. They have no "neuro." So we went to hospital B.

All of a sudden, a couple minutes before we got to hospital B, he perked up and became very alert. So IC [intracranial] bleed or hypoxia problem? He was 95 percent on room air, but his tidal volume was decreased and he had some wheezes. Big smoker. Later when I checked on him, they said he was "in and out." So it's probably a head problem.

Friday, 6-24-05, 8:47 a.m.
So, was it the beer that caused his stupidity or did it just intensify a preexisting lack of good judgment? Last night, a homeless thirty-four-year-old man went Dumpster diving for pizza for his "friends." He obviously didn't check his landing area first and cut his hand across the palm on some broken glass.

We picked him up at Serene and Eastern. FD already had his right hand wrapped in 4 x 4s and Kerlix, so we couldn't see it. I asked the fireman (so I didn't have to unwrap it to see) if a regular ER would be OK or if he needed to go to trauma. ER was OK.

He had been drinking a lot. He was obnoxious, foul mouthed most of the time, but would listen to me off and on. He didn't seem really intoxicated, just stupid, loud mouthed, and uncooperative.

We took him to hospital H because we were so close. Unfortunately, we had to wait awhile. Not a good thing. I lectured him, told him he needed stitches, but he wanted to leave. We took the IV out and unwrapped his hand so we could see and hopefully convince him he needed to stay. The laceration was about two inches long, didn't look too bad until you pulled it open. The lac went all through the fatty tissue. It had stopped bleeding. He was being such a pain in the ass we finally gave up and let him go.

Only a few minutes later, he walked into the lobby dripping blood all over the floor. Another medic and I rewrapped his hand. He was still being verbally combative and obnoxious, so hospital security called the police. But security ended up 86-ing him from property before they came.

He just wouldn't listen to me even though I was the only one he liked. In the truck (while we were still on scene), he started trying to feel my leg when I was taking his blood pressure. Metro told him to stop it. Then later, he said he would make love to me every night and rub my feet after I got off work. Only from the drunks...Oh, well.

Saturday, 6-25-05
Last night, I talked to another crew who ended up transporting our patient (man with lac on hand). He took his dressing off, again, and the laceration started bleeding in a convenience store. The crew found him lying down. His blood pressure was a little low and he didn't give them any problem.

Sunday, 7-15-07
Had a couple interesting calls recently.

Early in the morning, a petite eighty-five-year-old female was sleeping in her recliner. She said she thought she was having a dream that made her stand up suddenly, maybe got a little dizzy, and fell on the floor. She landed on her left hip.

When we got there, she was sitting on the floor next to the chair. Looking at her legs you could tell she either dislocated or fractured (or both) her hip (or upper femur). Usually, in these cases we put the patient on a scoop (metal, sometimes plastic, slightly concave board that comes apart lengthwise) to help pick them up. But she was so tiny we decided to Georgia street her. To do this, someone gets behind the patient, reaches around under their arms and grabs the patient's opposite wrist. Another person lifts the legs, usually at the knee. So, the fireman got behind our cute, little old lady and said, "Cross your arms." She said, "I already prayed!" I started laughing out loud. It was so cute and unexpected.

Sunday, 8-26-07, 5:52 p.m.
Wednesday night, we had a man who went roller-skating for the first time in ten years. He was with younger family members. He said he was just "cruising along" when his left leg went forward and his right leg went back. He dislocated his right ankle and fractured his fibula. The end of the tibia was medially protruding, skin intact. He didn't want any morphine. I asked him several times. He rated the pain initially only a 2/10. Before we left the trauma center, I asked him to sign my paperwork, but he was so "snowed" on pain medication they gave him that he couldn't do it.

Wednesday, 9-19-07, 5:35 a.m.
Last week, we had a call for a middle-aged man (not homeless looking) who was sleeping outside on Main Street near St. Vincent's. His wife and child were at Shade Tree nearby. A couple mean, punk, juvenile boys splashed acid (probably battery acid) on him and ran off. He had little spots of acid burns (looked like it was eating away at his skin) on both his forearms, a few on his shoulders, right side of his face, and a long wound on the left side of his neck.

When we pulled up, FD was rinsing his arms with water. We poured another bottle of saline irrigation on his arms and his neck. Hospital C is the burn center. I gave him 5 mg of morphine on the way in to start him on pain control. I'm sure he got plenty more at the hospital.

Thursday, 10-4-07, 5:03 p.m.
We got a call for a five-year-old boy who fell off his bunk bed and fractured his arm. He got up after his fall and got on his mom's bed. He was there for a little while until his mother heard his pain response and checked him out. When we got there he was...

Sunday, 10-7-07, 6:21 p.m.
(To continue)...lying on his back with his right arm next to his side. There was obvious deformity of his ulna just below his elbow. The ulna looked like it was about ready to poke through his skin (with the sharp tip pointing toward his hand). This little twenty-eight pound five-year-old was such a trooper! Not a moan...a cry...or

even an "ouch!"

When we got in the truck, I started an IV on his left hand. I wasn't going to give him any medication, so I let my partner be in back with him. After we took him to hospital C peds, I went back to the truck to look for a teddy bear. All the trucks used to have teddy bears to give to the little kids, but no luck tonight.

Sunday, 1-6-08, 5:32 p.m.

I've missed a lot of possibly interesting entries, but oh, well. I don't really feel like trying to catch up, but maybe I will mention a few weird calls.

A young woman was visiting a friend who lived near 28th and Bonanza. I remember that night was very windy for a while. These women went out for a while. When they returned home, they pulled the car into the driveway. Just as the visiting woman was stepping out of the passenger's side, a large branch from the tree overhead broke loose and fell, hitting her on the head and knocking her down to the ground. She was complaining mostly of back pain.

I was quite surprised when we pulled up. The tree in the yard was about forty feet tall! A large branch about eight to ten inches in diameter and about fifteen feet long broke off from a branch high up and crashed down landing on the house and the car and hitting the woman. What unfortunate timing!

Sunday, 2-17-08, 4:39 p.m.

Friday, we had an interesting day. We transported an older gentleman from a military retirement home to hospital O. He had an abscess on his buttocks that was responding to antibiotics. After transporting him, while we were at the hospital, we learned of a woman who needed to be transported. OK. So we told the staff we would take her as long as dispatch would agree. We had to wait one and a half hours because of all the insurance red tape for them to find her a bed in another hospital.

The woman, who is eighty-six years old, lives with her son. They have a rental house across the street from their house. She, obviously very independent, wanted to bring a bathroom door from across the street to her house. She pushed a dolly across the street, loaded the door on it, and headed back across the street.

It had been pretty windy (up to 67 mph the previous day) lately. While in the street, the wind caught the door, whipped it around hitting her on the right side of her head and knocking her down to the pavement. She said the next thing she knew, she was in an ambulance. Apparently, she had lost consciousness. I believe the ambulance crew was probably a volunteer crew. I don't know. She should have been put in a C-collar and on a backboard. There was definitely some potential for spinal injury there. It happened about 8:30 a.m.

Monday, 2-18-08, 5:18
(To continue) She had a CT scan done which showed an IC (intracranial) bleed on the left side of her head. They think it was a subarachnoid bleed. She was, obviously, complaining of a headache. Sometimes I wonder about clinics and some hospitals. She didn't have any oxygen on, they hadn't checked her C-spine, and still, after several hours, had no pain meds yet.

While we were waiting for all the red tape so we could transport our little old lady, a man came in with a finger injury. And this was another wind-related accident. The wind blew over a tree. The patient, in his forties, and another man were trying to put the tree (size? Don't know) on, I believe, the bed of a truck. The tree rolled toward the patient and a branch came around and landed on his right index finger. Quickly, without thinking, he yanked his hand out and the tip of the finger came off.

A woman came in with him and she had a baggie that contained the fingertip and some freezer ice things. I saw the X-ray and he had a nice clean chopped-off finger just barely past the last knuckle (closest to the finger tip). I think the tip was too crushed to save. The doctor just sewed the finger closed and he needs to go to a hand specialist.

Sunday, 3-30-08, 8:02 p.m.
We had a call to transport a forty-year-old man to hospital C to get a CT scan of his head. In February, he was assaulted at a bar and received a skull fracture and a subdural hematoma. He had to have a craniotomy and have the hematoma evacuated. His mental status has been affected. The nurse said he was tracking with his eyes and, per the paperwork, was obeying some commands (don't know to what extent). But they said lately he's gone downhill.

When we were with him initially, he would move his eyes a little when you called his name. And it looked like he was looking at you. I saw no movement of his arms or legs.

At hospital C, we had to wait for a while in the hallway. My partner and I were talking to him, believing he could understand, and trying to instill a positive attitude. "You will get better!"

After the CT scan, on the way back to his rehab, I asked my partner to play some music for him. I asked if he liked the music to blink his eyes for me. He did! I asked him a few other questions and he blinked his eyes in response. Did he want music played for him at rehab? Yes. I told him I would tell the nurse.

When we got to rehab, we put him back in bed. I was standing near the head of the bed on his left side and my partner was near his feet facing away from him toward the gurney. All of a sudden he started to raise his left hand. Wow! "Look, look!" I said to my partner. Then he started to raise his right arm, then his torso started to come up and it looked like he was trying to smile. That was so exciting! It really gave me an emotional lift. We told the nurse and she was pretty excited, too.

His father was there earlier. And his sister and mother. Keep on hoping. My partner and I tried to find a music channel on TV for him, but couldn't find anything good. I ran across *Scrubs* and asked if he liked that. He blinked his eyes "yes." So he started watching that. I really hope he gets better and becomes more like his normal self.

Monday, 8-4-08, 2:42 a.m.
Now for the "good" part. OK, let's see. What noteworthy patients have I had recently?

A 305-pound, five foot-nine inch woman got in an argument with a male friend of hers. He punched her in the face and she fell to the ground. When she got up, she heard a crack in her ankle. She was wearing sandals with soles about three inches thick. So she probably twisted her ankle on the way down. I asked her why she wore such thick soles and she told me the cushioning helped with her diabetic neuropathy. A bit overdone, huh? Well, she probably fractured her ankle. It was swollen and on the inner area there was a spot where blood was slowing dripping. I think the fractured bone was just underneath the skin with only a tip that poked through the skin.

Tuesday, 11-10-09, 6:29 p.m.

Last night at about 10:30, we got a call for a possible jumper, body on the freeway. We were posted at Tropicana and Koval. This person was supposedly under the Tropicana overpass and on I-15. As we approached the freeway, I could see the traffic backing up in the southbound lanes. So I told my partner (she was driving) to take the southbound on-ramp and we could oppose traffic for a short distance to get to the scene. The FD engine was already blocking traffic and the FD rescue and NHP [Nevada Highway Patrol] responded.

A man around forty years old was lying prone in the traffic lane. Pulseless, apneic, fixed dilated pupils. The skin behind his left knee was torn open laterally all the way across. He had closed deformity to his left arm and there was blood under his head. There were abrasions (minor) on his back and legs. His shoes and hat were on the pavement and he was wearing only socks and underwear.

A man standing nearby was talking to NHP because he hit the man. I missed most of the conversation, so I talked to him also. The driver couldn't tell me if the man fell from above or came from the side. I looked up and the flyover from the southbound exit to eastbound Tropicana was pretty much right above us. Why, why? It's so sad that people get to the point where they have no hope!

CHAPTER FOURTEEN

NO ORDINARY JOB

Friday, 5-30-03, 4:24 a.m.
Monday, my partner called off (she was moving that weekend) and Denise called me from the sup's office at about 1:30 p.m. (after four hours of sleep). She asked me if I wanted to work state line with her. Sure, give me an hour and I'll be there. So I worked from about 2:30 p.m. until 7:00 a.m. (state line shifts are twenty-four hours). We had free dinner at the hotel, ran two calls (canceled on both), then went back to their trailer for the duration. Until midnight, it was still holiday pay (Memorial Day—double time). Not too bad getting paid for sitting in a recliner watching TV, dozing off now and then.

Monday, 10-13-03, 3:57 a.m.
I think most of us would be surprised if we knew how we have affected the lives of other people. I worked an overtime shift tonight. We brought a patient to hospital A and had to sit in the hall, waiting with our patient, like several other crews. As I was writing my report someone said something that caught my attention. I looked up and asked what he was talking about. A young man, EMT I, sitting kitty-corner from me said I came to his grade school and did a presentation for career day. I brought the ambulance. My daughter was in his class. He remembers her. It was her fifth-grade class at Doris Reed Elementary School. He said it was because of me that he was working as an EMT. He said I was terrific.

I later called my daughter and she remembers him. I have a bunch of pictures from that day. I'm going to try to get ahold of him so I can give him a couple pictures.

Wednesday, 10-15-03, 10:59
Last night, about 2:30 a.m., I had a first in my eleven years working in this field. We had been working several hours already, transported someone to hospital J in Henderson, came back into town, and transported a patient to hospital B. We were in the hospital thirty to

forty-five minutes. My new partner's intern and I went outside to the truck. I got in the driver's seat and started to shut the door. Then I smelled a really strong odor. What is that? We got out, puzzled, looking around. I popped open the hood. Then the intern found the cause. There was a fire under the driver's seat! Between the seat cushion and the metal frame below was a horizontal space where you could see underneath. No doubt about it. There was fire under the seat.

The intern got the fire extinguisher from the oxygen cabinet behind the driver's door. He doused it a couple times. Then my partner looked behind the seat, smelled the same odor, and sprayed it one more time. We (I made her call this time because I called last night for a malfunctioning rear air conditioner) called the mechanic and he said to drive it back to the station and get a new truck. I called the sup and told him I wasn't comfortable driving it after what happened. He drove over with his sup intern. The intern ended up driving the truck back and we rode with the sup in his truck. Now, this is the second time I have had a fire on my ambulance. The first time, the front brakes lit on fire.

Comment: Someone told me that the mechanic believes the fire was caused by heavy people sitting in the driver's seat causing the supporting springs/wires to break. Then the broken wires damaged the electrical wiring under the seat.

Thursday, 11-13-03, 7:17 a.m.
It seems like a majority of the time at work we get posted downtown. It is the highest priority post. But most people don't like it because we get a lot of calls for drunk, homeless people in that area. When I see tourists walking around downtown, I think to myself, "Why are you in this area?" There are so many scurvy, run-down hotels/motels around here, especially on Fremont Street, hookers walking around, people buying/selling drugs.

Last night after we cleared from hospital B, we were very surprised to get posted at 27J, an indoor post at Flamingo and Jones. I quickly fell asleep in the reclining couch. The pager went off for an MVA [motor vehicle accident] near Sahara and Jones. When I looked at the clock in the ambulance, it was 4:35 a.m.! I slept longer at post than I did yesterday at home. Don't misunderstand, though, this doesn't happen very often.

Comment: The indoor posts (apartments, of which we had about six) are no more! Now we sit inside the trucks around the area of our given street intersections. Technically, we can go anywhere within a half-mile radius of that intersection. There are numerous posts around town. They are in strategically designated areas to help the trucks respond to 911 calls within the allowed response time. So now if I have any downtime, I can take a nap in the truck, sitting up, and get neck pain and a headache from the uncomfortable position. Wah! Right? Speaking of sleep, there are rules for sleeping at work. See the next entry.

Monday, 12-1-03, 10:49 a.m.
Did I mention the time a male nurse caught me taking a nap in the ambulance at hospital N? We were posted in that area, so I parked the truck toward the end of the driveway (near the ER). I fell asleep sitting there.

"Lynn, wake up!" My partner woke me up to see the nurse standing by my window. I was zonked out with my mouth wide open. How embarrassing! There are certain sleeping rules I try to follow at work. You have to sleep in a position so you don't mess your hair up (and get bedhead), get marks all over your face, mess up your mascara, snore too loudly. In other words, don't get too comfortable.

Wednesday, 12-31-03, 7:53 a.m.
Why, why, why are men so violent toward women? Yesterday morning, my partner told me that a nurse was killed in a domestic incident. Who, we didn't know. After asking around, found out that the nurse had a bad domestic fight with her boyfriend. Neighbors heard the noise and called Metro. Metro heard a gunshot when they got there. He shot and killed her, then killed himself.

Comment: I, of course, can't and don't want to mention any names, but too many people that I know in EMS have died. They include helicopter crash, motorcycle accident, couple suicides, aspiration while intoxicated, murder, several different medical reasons. It's always sad when someone dies while they are young.

Tuesday, 5-18-04, 9:36 a.m.

I worked an overtime shift on Saturday from 9:15 p.m. to 9:15 a.m. About 6:30 a.m., we had a call for chest pain. FD was there when we arrived. We went around to the back of the ambulance and opened the right back door. The left one wouldn't open. We fiddled with the locks. I even kicked the door from the inside while my partner tried opening it from the outside.

We went into the patient's house and I walked up to the fire medic and whispered, "We can't get our back door open." He and my partner went outside while I stayed inside and talked with the patient. They even got a tool from the rescue and tried to pry it open. They volunteered to transport the patient.

Tuesday, 6-7-05, 9:37 a.m.
Last night, Erin called me and asked if I would bake chocolate chocolate-chip cookies for her this morning. She made the dough, but knew she would be too tired to bake them. Too tired? Her? My whole body aches from being tired. Our first call last night, we transported a drunk man who fell and cut his head. We took him to hospital F. A cute fireman looked at me and said, "Hi, you look tired." Then at the end of the shift, sixteen calls later, someone in supply looked at me and said, "You look really tired." We transported only three people, but we made it on scene to eight other calls. Five others were canceled en route.

Yesterday morning, I went to a class about strokes. A lady from hospital A did the presentation. CVAs [cardiovascular accidents] interest me. I think my favorite calls are breathers, overdoses, unconscious/unresponsive, and unknown problem. I have never been too crazy about MVAs or chest pain. I think I don't like chest pain because frequently there is nothing you can see. You just have to go by what the patient says. Sometimes when a guy is suffering from incarceritis (the possibility, very real, of going to jail), he suddenly comes down with chest pain. BS! You have to treat most chest pain as legitimate, whether it's respiratory or cardiac, but sometimes you know it's a lie. Once, I had a tall, young man who was complaining of having angina after being detained by Metro. If you phrased the questions right, you caught him in his lie. He didn't like my questions and said he wanted a doctor. Sorry, buddy! Off to jail!

Tuesday, 3-14-06

Yesterday, I went to the store to fill my prescription for Zoloft (to help with my hot flashes—and I haven't had any bad ones since February 1). While I was waiting for the prescription to be filled, looking at the hair dye, I heard Tyler calling me. I'm still using the wheelchair because I have a circulatory problem in my left leg. Someone had passed out near the deli. I quickly wheeled over there.

About six employees were standing/sitting around a woman who was sitting on the floor, being propped up (she should have been lying down). She was awake, but appeared a little out of it, not saying much. I talked to a lady/employee near me, told her I was a paramedic. The patient didn't appear to be in dire distress and FD was on their way, so I wasn't too worried. Besides, what could I do without a blood pressure cuff, glucometer, and cardiac monitor? I went back over to get in line to pick up my pills. I really do miss my job. I got a little teary eyed.

Comment: After my accident on 10-17-05, I was off work until 6-5-07. After about August 2006, I started getting frustrated and depressed about the situation. I wanted to get back to work. Just had to be patient.

Wednesday, 9-19-07, 12:55 a.m.
Last week, I had the worst sore throat that I can remember. It was torture just to swallow my own saliva! Had a low-grade fever, too (99–100), but I wasn't sick enough to stay home. Thursday, I was tempted to call the sup and tell him I needed to go home. Just my luck, I did more telemetries than usual. On Friday, I did a tele (radio call) to hospital B. When I got there, two paramedics at the hospital who heard my telemetry said it sounded like Freddie Kruger and they were surprised it was me. My voice was really raspy, low, and gravelly.

Wednesday, 10-17-07, 10:26 a.m.
Oh, boy! Today is the second anniversary of my accident. So tonight, around 8:00 p.m., will be the approximate time. Last night, my partner and I got truck 63. It's one of the new Chevys. I heard that the siren on this one was weird, kind of like the supervisor truck's siren. To start the night out, we were posted downtown. We got a call at the Stratosphere. I was driving. When I flipped on the siren, both my partner and I jumped and then started laughing. The

siren sounded like it belonged on a spaceship. It's hard to describe, but it was a loud, lower pitched *woo-woo-woo* sound. By the time we got to the Stratosphere, tears were running down my cheeks because I was laughing so much. We ran a call later for an assault. Had to hold short. FD was already parked on the street corner. The firemen heard the sound before and they weren't sure what it was.

Comment: That *woo-woo-woo* sound is called the howler siren. Several of the ambulances have it. I have gotten used to it, so it doesn't seem weird anymore.

Sunday, 4-6-08
Friday, at work, I was driving the ambulance and was pulled over by Metro! We just got off the Decatur off-ramp from I-95 southbound. I heard a weird siren and my partner said Metro was behind us. So I figured I better pull over to get out of his way. Then a motorcycle cop pulled up to the driver's door. I recognized him. Seen him a zillion times. He just stopped us to tell us our right rear turn signal light was on. It was stuck on, not flashing. It has done that off and on. At the end of the shift I told the mechanic. He opened the electrical panel in the back and pounded on a few things. If it doesn't work right, hit it. Huh! It had already turned off again, but we'll see if it stays off now.

Wednesday, 12-3-08, 10:05 a.m.
Last Friday, my partner and I transported a patient (elderly male) to his home in Overton, NV. It's about eighty or so miles north of Las Vegas. After we dropped him off, we stopped at a convenience store to use the restroom and get a snack.

As usual, because they're a little heavy on my belt, I take my pager and scissors off before I use the toilet. I usually place them somewhere where I won't forget them. Well, got back to Las Vegas, next call...reached for my pager...it was not there! My pager and scissors were still in Overton. My partner thought that was funny.

I called Evan and he went to MapQuest on the computer and found the phone number for the store. I called that night and was told to call back on Monday and talk to the manager. She was very nice and said she would mail them (I asked if she could) to me, no charge. I did later send a money order to cover the cost, with a thank-you card.

When I got to work today, the box had arrived with my AWOL articles. I had received a page from the person in scheduling. She wanted to tell me they got a box for me that was beeping! I wonder if anyone in the post office noticed any beeping.

8-16-09

Last week, I was sitting in the ambulance at hospital B. One of the sups came over to my truck and said he needed to check the narcs. I figured he was checking for expired drugs and the log book. He found two morphine vials with broken seals.

Every night, I check to make sure the correct number of each drug is in the drug pouch. I guess I didn't notice the broken seal because it's not obvious without my reading glasses.

Thursday afternoon, I got a call from another sup telling me that I have to get drug tested within twenty-four hours because someone is tampering with the narcs. Later, I found out that 240 people have to get drug tested! My partner and I asked if we could go a few hours after we started our shift. It took almost two and a half hours.

They used test strips that showed immediately if you had some drugs in your body. My test came up nonnegative for benzodiazepines. That makes sense because I took half a Lortab and half a Soma in the morning to try to ease my back problem. Think I have a lumbar strain.

While we were at the quick care, a sup who was there said that anyone who tests nonnegative will probably be put on paid administrative leave until the lab (and management) verifies that they have prescriptions for the meds. So, tomorrow, I have to be ready to go to work, but can't until I'm cleared. Of course I'm not worried about the test because I would never tamper with the narcotics at work. Not only is it wrong, but it is completely stupid. And, besides, I have my own meds at home.

Thursday, 8-9-07, 7:16 a.m.

Tuesday night, we were on a call. I was driving Code 3 [life threatening] north on I-95 and exited the Lake Mead west off-ramp. It curves around and goes to Lake Mead going west back over the freeway. Just before the exit, we heard a strange noise from the engine. Coming into the curve I put on the brakes and they were really stiff. I don't like to swear much, but this was an "Oh, #!&#!!!"

moment. My partner thought I was kidding until I told her the brakes weren't working. I pushed harder on the brake pedal and it slowed down enough to make it around the curve. Next time, I'll use the emergency brake, too.

We called the sup and he told us to very carefully and slowly drive it back to the station. I drove the back streets going about 15 to 20 mph, and slowed down several yards before Stop signs and lights. It probably wasn't a smart thing for the sup to tell us to drive back with malfunctioning brakes, but if we didn't do it, he probably would. If I didn't think I could do it, I would have told him "No way!"

Friday, 12-31-10, 1:40 p.m.
New Year's Eve! Whoopee! Yesterday morning, I had a first at work. We ran a call on the Strip. We parked in back of the fire engine, which was facing north on the side of the Strip. We pulled out our gurney and walked over to where the patient was. We were very quickly canceled and went back to the truck.

I didn't notice when my partner closed the back door that it didn't shut evenly. We have been having problems with FD yanking on our back door latch, trying to open it when it's locked. They don't lock their rescue, but it is our company policy and my preference to keep the truck locked when we're not by it. Well, the bottom of the door was locked and the top was bent outward, not locked. Could not get the door open. So we had to lift up the gurney and put it through the side door! I have never done that before.

It was a little after 4:00 a.m. We had to go out of service and go back to the station. Because it was so close to Code 86 time [time to go back to the station to finish shift], we just finished our shift and hung out until clock-out time at 5:45 a.m. Last night, my partner put a sign near the door handle telling FD not to touch the door. They have damaged our door at least three times.

CHAPTER FIFTEEN

UNWRITTEN, BUT NOT FORGOTTEN

Saturday, 7-28-12, 2:04 p.m.

I officially started working for an ambulance company in October 1992. Due to no full-time openings, I worked part time for a year while I was still working full time as a bank teller. Finally, in January 1994, I got a full-time shift. Yeah!

Why did it take so long for me to start writing my journal? Guess it never occurred to me. In April 2003, I needed an outlet for my emotional frustrations. On 4-4-03 at 3:00 a.m. I grabbed a spiral notebook I had in my bedroom and wrote on the top of the first page: "My paper psychiatrist." Not that I really needed a psychiatrist! But writing down my thoughts and frustrations was kind of like talking to a shrink. Right? Except a lot cheaper!

About two weeks later, I made my first entry about a call I went on. And that's how it all started. Unfortunately, there are a lot of calls that weren't recorded in those first nine years, but some of them will definitely not be forgotten. I want to tell you about a few of them. Here goes.

This one is kind of gross and out of the ordinary and that is probably why I didn't forget it. I don't remember what year it was. We got a call at a trailer park on Tropicana. On our pager it said, "Dog ate her face." I knew this was going to be a weird one!

When we arrived at the trailer park, the fire department engine was parked in front of the trailer. As my partner and I were walking by the engine, the engineer was sitting in the driver's seat. He said, "You don't want to go in there! The dog ate her face!" My partner stopped in her tracks and opted not to go in, but I wasn't going to be grossed out. I think I can speak for some paramedics, including myself, that our curiosity to see the unusual is part of our nature.

When I entered the front door of the trailer, I saw a couple doggy treasures (poop!) on the floor. There was a quiet man sitting on the right end of the trailer. I assumed it was her husband. I went down a hallway to the left. At the end of the hallway was the bedroom.

Evidently, the woman was in the bedroom with the door closed when she died. And her little yap-yap dog (small furry dog) was in there with her. The woman was probably in her sixties, small, lying supine on the bed. Of course the dog got hungry after a while (assuming that was his motivation) and started chewing on her face. The lips and skin around her mouth and part of her lower cheek were gone. You could tell it had been a while since the dog had his "snack" because the edges were dry and curling under a little. Poor lady. Poor dog.

Let this next call be a lesson for anyone with a meth lab in their home. I believe the call came across as an explosion in the fireplace. My partner went in first. When he came running out I knew something was wrong! I had never seen him run before. He said we needed a backboard.

When I went in, I saw a lady lying on the living room floor with a sheet covering her. There was a man standing nearby. They had a meth lab in the house and there was an explosion. Her hand was blown off and all you could see were the ends of the radius and ulna sticking out at the end of her arm. I believe she also injured one of her feet.

Later I found out that she was a dancer. Career change. If I remember right, I believe her foot had to be amputated. She was a pretty lady. I was glad her face wasn't messed up.

Shortly after I became a paramedic (spring 1996), we were called to a rollover up north. I believe it was on I-95. I don't remember how far north it was, but the median was a large dirt area probably at least twenty to thirty feet wide. A car rolled over and a man was ejected and was lying in the dirt. We checked him out and he was dead. I remember one of the firemen looked at me and said, "You have the highest seniority. You have to call him." That basically means I had to officially say he is dead and that we are not going to resuscitate him. I did a quick mental "Gulp, aaaah!" and then said, "He's dead."

Then we heard a loud screeching of tires and looked to see a doofus who was coming from the other direction, who obviously wasn't paying attention and gawking at the accident scene, lose control of his car, do a 180, and land in the middle of the median. Fortunately, everyone in his car was OK.

In Nevada, there is a seat belt law for a good reason. People in EMS know better than almost anyone how good a law it is. Are you going to be ejected from a car if you have your seat belt on? Unlikely. I have told my children numerous times how dangerous it is to get in an accident without wearing your seat belt. I tell them I can think of only one call when it was fortunate that she didn't have her seat belt on. She was driving on a four-lane street, speed limit like 45 mph, got in an accident, and her car flipped over on its hood. It was a midsize car and while it was upside down, it looked like a convertible. I don't remember if it really was. The upper part of her body would probably have been mangled badly if she was restrained when it flipped. I don't believe she even went to the hospital. Lucky lady.

What happens when someone doesn't wear their seat belt? Here's a short list: young man's car rolls over and he is flung around in the car, breaks his neck, and he becomes a quadriplegic; man goes through the windshield; baby thrown out of van and dies; young lady takes her seat belt off for a second at a red light, the car is rear-ended and she dies. I could go on and on (and those were real people), but I think I made a point. Wear your seat belt!

I need to take a break and go to Walmart. More later.

Friday, 4-13-12, 5:05 p.m.

I talked with Denise last Saturday and she mentioned that she spoke with Calvin. He asked how I was doing. Denise said I was OK and that I was writing a book. She explained to him what it was about and he asked if I included the call we went on with the SIDS baby. I looked at all my notes and didn't find that call. How could I forget to write about that experience?

I started my journal entries in 2003. I was taking classes in 1992, with my official hire date as an EMT in October 1992. I went on several ride-alongs with an ambulance crew before I actually worked as an EMT. My first ride-along was one I will never forget. The first call was for a man at a casino who had a seizure. Nothing noteworthy about that. But the last call really hit me hard. I remembered the call, but because I never wrote it down in a journal, many of the details are lost. I called Calvin and talked with him about it and he gave me information I either forgot or never knew.

What I remember is going into the house and seeing a fifteen-month-old baby in the middle of the living room floor. Calvin did mouth-to-mouth ventilations for a few seconds, but there was nothing we could do for the baby. The father was sitting in a chair off to the side, very quiet. The wife was at work. Someone called her and told her she needed to come home. When she got home, she grabbed the baby and sat down in a chair, rocking the baby and crying hysterically. I remember seeing a lady on scene (presumably her friend) who I recognized from my grocery store. I had never seen a dead person before. And to make it worse, it was a poor little baby. It was a very emotional scene. I started to lose control. I went outside to cry. I still had young children (three to nine years old), so this was especially painful.

After speaking with Calvin, he told me the father handed him the baby when we arrived. The baby had been sick, saw a doctor, and was on medications. There was also a two-and-a-half-year-old child. The father said, "What am I going to tell my wife?" He felt so guilty. When the wife arrived, Calvin saw her outside the window, looking at the rescue. "Where's my baby? Where's my baby?" The mother was given Valium to help her calm down a little.

Calvin said until his daughter was three, he checked every night to see if she was OK. I think I was worse. I checked all four of my kids for years. I looked at their chests when they were sleeping to make sure they were breathing. Being a paramedic has made me more paranoid and worried about my children. My eyes have been opened to some of the terrible possibilities. Ever heard the saying "Ignorance is bliss"? It really is true in some cases.

For three days after that call, it really still bothered me. It haunted me and several times it still made me cry. And then something weird happened. All of a sudden, on the fourth day when I woke up, I was fine.

That was the first, but not the last time I shed tears on a call. It doesn't happen very often, fortunately. I realized after I spoke with Denise and Calvin that there were many "good" calls I didn't record between 1992 and 2003. Most of the memories are probably lost to me forever.

Monday, 8-27-12, 8:33 p.m.
Tuesday, I spent about six hours looking for my wallet. I really think my granddaughter took it off the kitchen counter (I know, I shouldn't have left it there!) and hid it. Finally, I found it on Thursday when I was going through my laundry basket to separate clothes for

washing. My granddaughter loves to take things and hide them somewhere in the house. It can be very frustrating.

During the six hours I was looking, I came across a letter that one of my supervisors wrote. Sometime back in 1998, I ran a call for an elderly woman who was having chest pain. On the way to the hospital, we talked about her upcoming move to another location. She said her husband has health problems, so he couldn't help much with the move. Sometimes, I really feel bad about my patients' situations. Most of the time, there is nothing I can do to help but talk with them. This time, I felt moved to help her. Until now, I forgot about the letter my supervisor wrote. This is what he wrote:

> This letter is to commend you on your performance and compassion shown toward an elderly couple that you met while performing your duties as a paramedic. You definitely went the extra mile and identified this couple's need for help with a move to a new residence on May 9, 1998.
>
> You and the group of volunteers you organized for the move are to be commended. Each of you should feel proud of a job well done. This was a situation extremely well handled and in my opinion an excellent example to all of us.
>
> I am impressed with your dedication for coming in on your day off to help them move. You are a great asset and I am proud to be associated with you.
>
> Sincerely [signed by my field supervisor]

I am not mentioning this event to pat myself on the back. And I'm sure I am not the only one who has gone the extra mile for one of their patients. Most of the time, we don't have the opportunity. We show we care by treating our patients with respect, helping them to feel more comfortable in their time of need, and giving them the best medical treatment possible. To be a good paramedic doesn't involve just having a lot of knowledge about paramedicine. Bedside manner is very important.

Yesterday (8-24-15) I read through this book, checking, for the last time, for any mistakes or things I wanted to change. It seems that no matter how many times I read through it, there is something I need to change. I sent it to a professional editor which helped a lot. It still may have some boo-boos. So be it! But this morning there were several calls that popped into my mind that never were recorded. I am going to describe them briefly, since most of the details are lost forever.

Many years ago we received a call for a man who stabbed himself. When we got to his apartment, he was on the kitchen floor. He had stabbed and cut himself numerous times. He stabbed himself twice in the stomach, and cut both wrists and his neck. Fortunately, the laceration to his neck did not penetrate his trachea. There was a lot of blood! We transported him Code 3 to hospital C trauma. On the way to the hospital we found out he did this because he found out he had AIDS! There was a female (relative, friend?) riding up front in the passenger's seat who was yelling at my partner, who was driving. "You're not driving fast enough! You're killing him!"

The next one was many years ago, also. Had a call for a man who was hit by a train in the northeast part of town (it was dark outside). The man was lying on the train tracks. When the engineer saw him, he blasted his whistle and the man lifted up his head. The engineer could not stop the train in time. We found the man underneath the train, several compartments down. We could see his intestines hanging out. I walked up to the front of the train and could see some hair stuck to the cow catcher (don't know the real name). Alongside the train tracks were little globules of fatty tissue. I thought it was strange that there were playing cards scattered down the train tracks, also.

I will never forget one of the shortest calls I ever had. We received a call for a person with a breathing problem. When we got on scene there was a man standing outside waiting for us. He walked up to the ambulance. One look at him and I could tell he had a serious problem. He was in respiratory distress. Serious distress! We immediately got him into the ambulance, put him on oxygen, and checked his blood pressure. His blood pressure was 300/200! Highest blood pressure I have ever seen. Those were the days when we used a manual blood pressure cuff. The top number didn't go above 300. I don't think we waited on scene with him. His lungs were full of fluid. I don't remember, but he most likely had a history of congestive heart failure. Everything was done en route to the hospital. I don't remember if I had time to do everything I wanted to do, which would have included, also, an IV, high dose nitro, and Lasix. I called the hospital on the radio to help them prepare for his arrival. From the time we got the call to the time we arrived at the hospital was only 11 minutes!

One more. This call was pretty recent. Another ambulance was called to the scene of an accident. A man driving a car hit a man on a scooter three times. The scooter man was inside the ambulance and was going to be transported. FD had checked out the man in the car and told the ambulance crew that he was OK. The female crew member stepped outside to talk to the man from the car. She soon realized that he was very confused. She took him over to their ambulance and started to check him out. His blood sugar was over 300. Due to his confused state and his elevated blood sugar, another ambulance crew was called to transport him. That would be me and my partner. When we pulled up he was sitting inside the side door of the ambulance. An IV had already been started. We put him on our gurney and took him over to our truck. He was definitely confused! He couldn't answer any questions appropriately. I decided to put him on a 3 lead EKG. It didn't look right. So I put him on a 12 lead. He was having a heart attack, what is called a STEMI (ST elevation MI). I asked him if he was having any pain. No. I think he was too confused to even answer that appropriately. Off we went to the hospital, Code 3, treating him for an MI. As usual, I did a radio telemetry to the hospital. After we arrived at the hospital, I was almost expecting my suspicions (of a heart attack) to be wrong. But the hospital agreed with me. Their question was how do you treat, or how much treatment do you give to someone who is so confused. I'm assuming they did what they needed to do.

CHAPTER SIXTEEN

TYPICAL PARAMEDIC, TYPICAL DAY

Just like most jobs, paramedics are all very different people. But if I had to describe a "typical" paramedic I would say male in his twenties to early thirties, outgoing, uses "colorful" language, enjoys a night out drinking, intelligent, attractive…But we're not all like that. There are many female paramedics. And some of us are a bit older. Take me, for example. I turned fifty-nine a couple weeks ago. I didn't start this career until I was thirty-nine. Before that, I spent about twelve years being a bank teller. Got so sick of that I had to do something completely different. Found it!

I have four grown children and two little grandchildren [now 3, as of October 2014]. I don't smoke, drink, or use drugs. Or swear very much. I can have fun without all that. But there were a few times when I was working that I let a few four-letter words escape.

Being a paramedic is really an eye-opener! We see the worst and sometimes the best side of the human race. I'm not talking just about blood and gore. We see the agony and misery that people have in their lives. Fortunately…My daughter just came in to tell me that my dog is stupid. And then she handed me a spatula with brownie batter on it. She's making brownies! It's a mix, but who cares! Need to take a break and enjoy my batter…

OK, I'm back. That was good. Have you ever read the comment on the box of cake mix that says "Do not eat raw cake batter"? Give me a break! Do you think we are stupid? Of course we shouldn't eat it. But most people taste a little bit, right? Back to what I was saying. Fortunately, we have our funny moments and our moments of joy we get to share with our patients.

I remember a couple times I had a patient serenade me all the way to the hospital. And the drunk men—they can be funny. "If I stopped using heroin would you go out with me?" "How about if I cut off my beard?" And they can be entertaining, too. They can say the silliest things.

Sorry. Let's get back to the topic. Now, what is a typical

workday like? I worked graveyard almost exclusively, so this will be from a night owl's point of view. I try to arrive about fifteen minutes prior to my scheduled time that my shift starts. We clock in using the wall phone. The supply department has a counter where they hand out the equipment we need to take to our trucks. Now, that includes a handheld radio, our computer, truck keys, and gloves. The paramedics get their narcotics from a special safe. Most of the equipment is already on the ambulance.

I believe that nobody is perfect and that includes the supply people. That is why I check out the equipment in the truck before we go available. If something is missing and we didn't know it, it becomes our problem and our patient's problem on a call.

When we go on a call, we have three basic pieces of equipment that we bring with us. That includes a cardiac monitor, portable oxygen tank, and a jump bag. And the gurney, of course! In this jump bag we have IV start kit, IV setups, medications, IO kit, oxygen masks, intubation kit, glucometer, and a few other things. I especially like to double-check the jump bag to make sure everything is in it. We are also supposed to check the truck oil.

After the truck is checked out, we are ready to go available. Dispatch is contacted on the truck radio and they assign us a post. A post is somewhere in town where they send us to wait for a call in that area. It is designated by the intersection of two streets. So we sit there and wait until someone calls 911. Normally, we keep the truck running. When it's one hundred degrees in the summer, there is no way we are going to turn off the truck! And it can get a little chilly at night during the winter.

One of the things I really enjoy about being a paramedic is that every day is different. And you never know what the day will be like. You never know what kind of calls you will get. When you are sitting in certain areas of town, some calls are more likely than others. But still, there is a lot of variety. Some of the most common types of calls are abdominal pain, breathing problem, chest pain, assault, fall, sick person, car accident, seizure, psych patient, intoxicated person, and traumatic injuries. And then there are some really weird ones. Those are the ones when you say to yourself, "You have got to be kidding me!"

After many years, and seeing many patients, I like to try to guess what's wrong with the patient before I get on scene. We receive the information for the call on the truck computer and also on our pagers. The information is limited, so I like to do a little guessing sometimes. For example, when we get a call, the information on our pager includes the following: run number (number assigned to the call), our medic number, call priority (Code 2 or 3), location on map book, address, type of call, and a short description of patient's complaint. If I got a call for a twenty-year-old female with breathing problem and numbness, my first thought is hyperventilation syndrome. On the way to the call, my partner and I often talk back and forth about what we think the call might be.

Just because someone calls 911 doesn't mean that they will go to the hospital. Sometimes, a patient will decide not to go. As long as they are alert and oriented, we can't force them to go. That would be kidnapping. There are so many times when we have to help them with their decision.

After we transport a patient to the hospital and our report is finished, we tell dispatch that we are available. Then they assign us to another post. And we wait again.

I remember one night I was working with a guy who now works for the fire department. We sat all night long and never got a single call. Not one! What a long, boring night.

Sometimes, there are nights when it's hard to find time to use the restroom or get something to eat. We don't get a lunch hour. Just eat when we can. And at night it is sometimes hard to find a restroom. When all the restaurants are closed we have to resort to convenience stores or casinos. I remember one night we drove to four different convenience stores looking for a restroom we could use. Usually the clerks are very nice to us. I don't know if they realize how much we appreciate their hospitality, especially at night!

It's hard to say how many calls we would get on a typical night. It might be eight calls with four transports, or it could be thirteen calls with six transports.

Comment: **Friday, 11-14-2014, 9:49 p.m.** Earlier, I was reading a Yahoo report about a woman who died possibly from eating commercial raw cookie batter infected with *E. coli*. I also read some articles online about the risk of raw eggs carrying salmonella. The very young and elderly are most at risk for serious complications. Excuse me for my sarcasm a couple pages back. I understand the potential risks, even though they are very small. I definitely do not eat undercooked meat!

CHAPTER SEVENTEEN

A BIT OF THIS AND THAT

This is the chapter where I get to say whatever I want to all of you. Just remember, my comments are not to be taken as medical or legal advice. I am just expressing my opinions. And I'm sure some of the things I bring up are a concern or a pet peeve to other paramedics.

Imagine you are driving and you pull over to the right for the ambulance that has its lights and siren on. Then you see it go through the intersection. Right after it gets through the intersection, the lights and siren turn off and it pulls into the 7–Eleven. What? They went Code 3 to get a soda? No. We receive many calls at convenience stores. Maybe that's where the patient is. Many times while we are driving to a call, we get canceled. If we're already going through an intersection, we'll shut down on the other side. If we pull into a 7–Eleven, there may be a good reason. Dispatch still hasn't told us where to go; I have really needed to use a restroom for the last hour and if I don't go now, I feel like I am going to POP; I really need a snack—I think my blood sugar is getting low; I'm thirsty…

Please pull to the RIGHT and then stop when you see an emergency vehicle with lights and siren on. Don't panic and stop in front of us! If you're sitting at a red light when you see our lights, DO NOT go through the red light to get out of our way. If you are in the middle of the intersection when you see us, do not slam on the brakes. We don't want any accidents or want anyone getting hurt on our way to the call.

For anyone with a lot of medical problems or someone who takes a lot of medications, there is something you can do that will help us a lot. Make a list of all your health problems, medications you take, and any allergies you may have to medications. When we come to your home, you can give us the list. That helps SO much.

Do not be afraid to call 911 if you have a medical problem. You know when something is not normal for you. We will come and check you out and help you decide if you need to go to the hospital.

One thing that really ruffles my feathers is the paramedic (usually the fire department) that says you HAVE to go to the hospital, or if you call us back later, then you HAVE to go. I can't remember how many times I have been on scene and heard those words. As long as a patient is alert and oriented, or is not a danger to him-/herself or anyone else, he/she can refuse transport.

It's after 11:00 p.m. and I have to get up at 6:00 to pick up my grandkids. I can't watch those two when I'm too tired. That makes for a miserable day. More later…

OK, next day.

As a paramedic, my primary concern is to treat my patient's medical problem. There are times when financial situations should be considered. Say, for example, a person has a sore on his foot that isn't healing. He is a diabetic and has had the sore for several months (had this type of call several times). He calls 911 because it hurts and he's tired of the pain. We ask patients for their picture ID and insurance card(s). Then the thought goes through my mind: Should I be nice to this man or just say, "OK, let's go"? He has no insurance and I'm compassionate tonight, so I give him the options: take the ambulance to the hospital, have someone drive you, go to a quick care, or see your own doctor tomorrow. For a medical problem that is not emergent, there may be better options than taking an ambulance.

DO NOT go to quick care if you are having chest pain or trouble breathing. If you're out and about and the quick care is right there, go for it! Otherwise, please call 911. We will be there quickly and start the treatment you need. If you go to a quick care, you will get treatment, but then they will call an ambulance to take you to the hospital. An extra bill you don't need. Quick cares have value—been there, done that for myself and my children—but not for anything serious.

Do not take prescription medications that are not prescribed for you. The average person doesn't know "Is this medication right for my problem?"; "Will it interact with my other meds?"; "What are the side effects?"; "How much should I take?"; "What are the contraindications?"

When your seriously sick loved one is being transported to the hospital by ambulance and you are following in your car, DO NOT try to keep up with the ambulance if it is traveling with lights and siren. You might get stopped by the police or get in an accident.

If you're out partying in Las Vegas, do not leave your drink unattended. Do not accept a drink from a stranger. Some idiots like to put drugs in people's drinks.

When you're visiting Las Vegas in the summer, drink water! Don't want you to ruin your fun!

Do not go off your prescribed medications without talking with your doctor. And please, all of you with high blood pressure or diabetes, take your condition seriously. If you run out of your meds, get them refilled quickly. If money is a problem, talk to a social worker, get Medicaid, borrow money, do anything (that's legal) to get your meds. The possible consequences of not having your meds are scary.

Do not jaywalk! I remember a call I had years ago for an auto-ped on Tropicana. An elderly couple was jaywalking. The husband was hit and thrown about sixty feet. Sad, sad! I walked with the wife to the casino nearby so she could be with her friends. I was doing OK until she started talking to her friends. So tragic! I excused myself and left with tears in my eyes.

DO NOT DRINK AND DRIVE! No excuse. I can't stress that enough. Drunk drivers kill.

If you drink too much, can't take care of yourself, or pass out, you may wake up in the hospital.

Someday soon, I will hang up my stethoscope and say good-bye to a worthwhile and fulfilling career. I thank ALL my patients who have made it an unforgettable experience.

So, if anyone asks me what I have been doing for a living for the past twenty-plus years, I can tell them that I have been hanging around on STREET CORNERS, picking up STRANGERS, and pushing DRUGS!

www.ingramcontent.com/pod-product-compliance
Lightning Source LLC
Chambersburg PA
CBHW070812180526
45168CB00002B/593